D1285463

DEADLY DOCTRINE

Caution—Christianity may be hazardous to your health!

DEADLY DOCTRINE

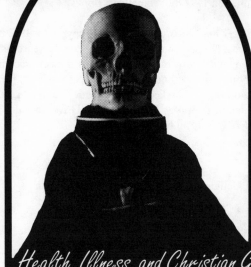

Health, Illness, and Christian God-Talk
Wendell W. Watters, M.D.

PROMETHEUS BOOKS • BUFFALO, NEW YORK

This book is dedicated to all those who choose to think for themselves on existential issues, no matter how lonely and painful that may be.

Published 1992 by Prometheus Books

96 95 94 93 92   5 4 3 2 1

Library of Congress Cataloging-in-Publication Data

Watters, Wendell W.
    Deadly doctrine : health, illness, and Christian god-talk / by Wendell W. Watters.
        p.   cm.
    Includes bibliographical references and index.
    ISBN 0-87975-782-5
    1. Christianity—Controversial literature. 2. Health—Religious aspects—Christianity. 3. Mental health—Religious aspects—Christianity. I. Title.
BL2775.2.W27   1992
261.8'321—dc20   92-29838
                                                                       CIP

Printed in the United States of America on acid-free paper.

"If people were a little more ignorant, astrology would flourish—if a little more enlightened, religion would perish."

—Robert G. Ingersoll

Contents

Introduction

Churchgoers who are committed believers may be offended by this book, if, indeed, they read it at all. People who are atheists, freethinkers, or humanists (who comprise approximately one-fifth to one-quarter of the world's population)[1] may find much to help them in their never-ending quest for genuine meaning in their lives. I have written primarily for those who, while nominally religious, are increasingly dissatisfied with the theistic orientation to life, and, in spite of the guilt they are encouraged to feel for doubting, are prepared to explore the humanistic alternative.

Religion is an existential soother to which individuals, having been born atheists, are encouraged to become addicted as they grow up in our theistic society. Christianity is the pacifier *par excellence,* claiming to alleviate cosmological fears—fears largely of its own creation—and to relieve guilt that has been stimulated in the believer by Christian god-talk. In order to sell their product, god-talking salesmen do everything possible to prevent the believer from growing up emotionally and psychologically, manipulating the greedy egocentric infant in us all with preposterous promises of eternal bliss in the hereafter.

In our addiction, we tend to lose sight of the price tage carried by most drugs, some higher than others. Heroin, which eases the suffering of the patient in severe pain, is also the direct cause of much human misery, with addiction linked to widespread criminal activity. Alcohol is used as a social lubricant, enlivening many an otherwise dull gathering; but it also contributes to most of the carnage on our highways and produces untold suffering for victims and their families. Smoking was once considered a routine feature of "adult" behavior; addiction to nicotene is now known to be the cause of many serious

9

obstetrical, cardiac, and respiratory problems, both in the addicts themselves and in those around them.

The thesis of this book, based on many years of clinical experience, is that, despite the so-called comfort of the Christian message, Christian doctrine and teachings, deeply engrained as they are in Western society, are incompatible with the development and maintenance of sound health, and not only "mental" health, in human beings. It has been painful for all of us who enjoy the benefits of this technological age to tolerate the fact that the air we breathe contains industrial pollutants capable of causing lung cancer, and that many of the foods we eat contain additives that are harmful to human health in a variety of ways. Similarly, Christians will find it difficult to entertain the notion that the tenets of their faith (one many claim to be as essential as food and air) have side effects that are deleterious to their health and that of their children. Simply put, Christian indoctrination is a form of mental and emotional abuse that can adversely affect bodily health in the same way a drug can.

On the social level, the history of Christianity does not make for pleasant reading, once the reader gets below the self-serving veneer glued to that history by centuries of Christian historians. It is remarkable that anyone can read that record, even in its whitewashed version, and still remain a practicing Christian. The highlights of that chronicle are all too familiar: the bizarre debauchery and bloody deeds of the viciously corrupt medieval popes; four centuries of absolute madness during the Crusades, in which millions of Christians, Jews, and Muslims were slaughtered or starved; six centuries of terror perpetrated by the Roman and Universal Inquisition, also called "The Holy Office" (not abolished until 1965), during which countless thousands of human beings were imprisoned, tortured, or burned at the stake; the censorship, imprisonment, or martyrdom endured by Galileo, Bruno, and other scientists who challenged biblical "truths" by daring to use human reason in an attempt to make sense of the universe; and the burning at the stake of thousands of women and young girls during the great witch-hunting mania. And all in the name of Jesus Christ, Son of God and Savior of the World.

Christian god-talkers have an ingenious explanation for this mad, bloody record: to wit, these dreadful events were really manifestations of Satan working in human beings (alas, even in holy men), and thus they constitute additional proof of man's innate evil as well as provide further evidence of the need for God's divine guidance and grace through Jesus Christ. However, this explanation ignores the fact that most of these deeds were carried out *in the name of* Jesus Christ; they were relentlessly logical outcomes of the core doctrine of Christianity. Yet we are asked by Christian god-talkers to believe quite otherwise and, in fact, to embrace that doctrine more completely and more faithfully; it is rather like trying to douse a fire with gasoline.

We should not delude ourselves into believing that these foul deeds are confined to past centuries; our own age has borne witness to the Nazi holocaust and the horror of Jonestown. Christians want to believe that Jim Jones was mad and that the Nazis were the enemies of Christianity, pointing to Hitler's harsh treatment of many Christian clerics as evidence to support that contention. But it was not Jim Jones's madness that made nine hundred people follow him to the Guyana jungle looking for salvation; it was society's readiness to find this sort of thing not only acceptable but even admirable. As for the Nazis, we seem to forget that they all learned their fanatical anti-Semitism from their Christian parents and nannies. Hitler was an altar boy in his youth; in his book *Mein Kampf*, he made frequent references to the Lord and His abomination of the Jews. Tom Harpur, an Anglican priest-turned-writer but a practicing Christian still, has written: "Though it has taken decades since the event, Christian theologians now recognize the full extent of Christian complicity in the Holocaust of roughly six million Jews by the Nazis."[2]

This book does not deal with the machinations of Christian doctrine on the social level, however; readers interested in the possible relationship between religious belief and man's inhumanity to man (and to woman) on a social, global level are referred elsewhere.[3]

Nevertheless, the bloody legacy of Christianity to the history of Western culture is directly relevant to my argument in this book, for it represents one attempt to make sense out of clinical observations made over a twenty-five year career as a psychiatrist working with individuals, couples, and families who have manifested a wide range of psychiatric, emotional, and interpersonal problems.* As existing theoretical models of human behavior (psychoanalysis, systems theory, and learning theory, for example) reached the limits of their explanatory power, I was moved to go beyond these conceptual approaches and to examine our society itself in order to determine the lessons people learn about life from its structural givens, as well as what they pick up in the cultural nourishment they assimilate. It soon became evident that in the social woodwork of the Western world, the cross of Jesus Christ had been carved deeply over the past two thousand years, and that even people who never darkened a church door were strongly affected by many teachings of Christianity, often without even knowing it.

This book is written in the hope that it will stimulate others interested in human well-being to explore further the thesis that those social attitudes derived directly or indirectly from Christian doctrine are incompatible with healthy human development. Despite seven years of personal analysis, my training as a psychoanalyst, and a quarter century of experience as a psychiatrist,

---

*My patients have led me to the conclusions I have reached about the hitherto unrecognized role of Christianity in people's lives.

this was a difficult issue for me to pursue. My early upbringing was in the Anglican (Episcopalian) faith, and many of the messages emanating from that institution still reverberate at some level of my being. From the dimly re-membered past come the words of Second Peter, Chapter II, Verse 1: "But there were false prophets also among my people, even as there shall be false prophets among you, who privily shall bring upon themselves quick destruc-tion." There is some truth to the old saying, "You can take the boy out of the church, but you cannot take the church out of the boy who continues to live inside the man."

Evidence that religion is irrelevant would not move me to write a book; there are already many excellent works on that topic. However, evidence that religion is not only irrelevant but actually harmful to human beings should be of interest, not only to other behavioral scientists, but to anyone who finds it difficult to live an unexamined life. Finally, the argument advanced in this volume should stir the political decision makers, who complain about the high cost of health care even while continuing to subsidize that very institution that may be actually making the public "sick."

Traditional believers tend to cling to their religious systems with a tenacity not demonstrated in the area of scientific research. Addictive belief systems become so much a part of the identity of some people, that it is often impossible to determine where the individual being stops and the religious group-think starts. At the same time, the humanity of other believers has not been completely stifled by their religious indoctrination; and I consider many in this group to be my friends. I earnestly hope that our personal relationship is strong enough to withstand the possibly alienating effect of this book, that the strength of the human bond we share will enable us to agree to disagree about existential matters.

NOTES

1. *Humanist Association of Canada Newsletter* (Spring 1992) (from figures taken from the *Encyclopedia Britannica Book of the Year,* 1989).

2. Tom Harpur, *For Christ's Sake* (Toronto: Oxford University Press, 1986), p. 9.

3. Charles W. Sutherland, *Disciples of Destruction* (Buffalo, N.Y.: Prometheus Books, 1987).

1

Health and Christian Doctrine:
Framing the Hypothesis

"It is clear that our values make a big contribution to disturbances in early childhood."

—Jules Henry (1972)[1]

"We have not yet learned to be entirely secular, and continue to reproduce Christian patterns of thought and behaviour in secular ways."

—Karen Armstrong (1986)[2]

In all human cultures, in all ages, the state of "being ill" has been associated with fear and superstition, each culture developing its own causal explanations for the various illness states as well as its own treatments and "cures." Such explanations were always reflections of that culture's religious beliefs, ecological concerns, and its stage of economic and scientific development. Until recently, such explanations assumed a simplistic linear causality: the sufferer was sick because of bad air inhaled through the lungs, or other noxious agents, natural or supernatural, ingested by mouth; or else he or she had violated a tribal taboo, or sinned against a god and was being punished by the relevant deity. With the invention of the microscope and the discovery of bacteria, an important step in the evolution of modern medicine, hopes ran high that all human illness would eventually be cured, a hope encouraged by the discovery of antibiotics.

We now know that things are not that simple. Often the form and intensity of an illness is strongly influenced by the individual's psychological attitudes and behavioral responses to the physical symptoms, whatever their immediate "cause." The actual, overt expression of symptoms is determined by a complex circular pattern of interactions among various levels of functioning, notably the physiological (biological), the affective (emotional), the cognitive (thinking, attitudinal), and the behavioral (what the individual does in response to the interacting events on the other levels). An example of this interaction is a situation in which, in a moment of intense physical and emotional activity, an individual sustains an injury, the pain of which does not register subjectively until the intense emotional and physical activity subsides. Whether the process begins in a specific lesion or is the end result of a stressful conflictual situation, it is the overall behavioral response of the patient—the "illness behavior"—that influences the reactions of others (i.e., the family and the health care system) to the "sick" individual.

A "lesion," first of all, is an anatomical abnormality, such as a broken leg, an inflamed joint, a tumor, or a diseased heart valve. "Stress" is the term applied to situations in which the individual's psychobiological mechanisms are overwhelmed by psychological conflict or by severe challenges to that individual's coping capacity. Some lesions, e.g., poliomyelitis or cancer, may be totally unrelated to stress and caused by factors outside the influence of the adaptive capacity of the sufferer.* Other lesions, e.g., malignant tumors, are likely to constitute a stress to which the individual must adapt in one way or another. Conversely, certain states of chronic intense stress may engender hormonal and other biochemical imbalances, some without producing a lesion that can be identified by the pathologist, while other stress-related illnesses, such as peptic ulcers, eventually progress to the point where a true lesion is produced.

The term "illness behavior" applies to the sufferer's overall responses to symptoms, regardless of their origin. These behavioral responses are determined largely by the *meaning* this experience holds for the individual. David Mechanic refers to illness behavior in these terms: "The concept of illness refers to objective symptoms and their interrelations; illness behavior, in contrast, refers to the varying perceptions, thoughts, feelings, and acts affecting the personal and social meaning of symptoms, illness, disabilities, and their consequences."[3] At times, maximizing the overall response to symptoms may allow the individual to regress, to retreat temporarily from an adaptational challenge in some area of life such as occupation or relationships. If a parent or partner tends to be much more caring and affectionate in the presence of illness, the sufferer's response to it may be quite different than if the family is intolerant of illness

---

*Some would argue here that internal factors, such as the state of the individual's immune system, can be influenced by stress, but that is a more subtle level than the one on which we are operating at the moment.

in any form. In difficult life situations, minimal subjective symptoms may be associated with maximal objective illness behavior; the child who is anxious about going to school may somatize this anxiety in the form of a stomach ache, the pain of which becomes magnified in order to avoid the anxiety-producing situation, namely, going to school. Conversely, certain people may tend to deny the existence of symptoms and stoically minimize illness behavior to the point where they do not take appropriate steps to get needed medical aid.

Throughout this book we will be examining links between Christian doctrine and human suffering. We shall see that many aspects of Christian doctrine and teachings produce attitudes in care-giving adults that seriously compromise the adaptive growth of the child, resulting in severe conflict contributing to stress, both intrapsychically and interpersonally. This in turn may compromise the child's ability to cope with external stresses.

Mechanic has stated that "illness perception and response may be socially learned patterns developed early in life as a result of exposure to particular cultural styles, ethnic values, or sexual socialization; or they may result from a person's earlier experiences with illness; or they may be shaped by particular motivations, situational factors, or adaptive needs when symptoms or disability actually occur."[4] Whether one views religious socialization as a component of "cultural style" or "particular motivation," it certainly deserves its own place on Mechanic's list of determinants of illness behavior.

The possibility of an etiological connection between doctrinal Christianity and illness is not an idea that will be readily entertained, given the popular (mis)conception of the complementary nature of the role of the cleric and the health worker. Both are supposed to help people with their existential human concerns, whether these concerns are expressed "physically," "psychologically," or "spiritually." Many people are inclined to the view that there is a positive connection between faith and healing. Did not Jesus heal the sick? Was not Luke, one of his disciples, a physician? The truth is, however, that the connection between faith and healing has never been documented in any scientific study;[5] indeed, faith healing has been roundly discredited by the famed debunker of the paranormal, James Randi.[6]

Most health workers would rather not confront the distinction between themselves and their religious confrères. The health worker is or should be operating from a scientific perspective, whereas the cleric is operating from one that is antithetical to science. Charles Glock and Rodney Stark, in their book *Religion and Society in Tension,* contend that there is a "degree of wishful thinking" in the view that religious and scientific approaches to human behavior are complementary. They go so far as to state, "The seeming rapprochement between the natural sciences and religion has tended to obscure a growing tension between religion and the social sciences."[7] Since health care education has moved away from a narrow preoccupation with the natural, biological sciences, and become more involved in the social and behavioral sciences, thus encroaching on territory previously considered the turf of the god-talkers, this tension is bound to increase.

Family physicians and other primary health care professionals tend to agree that the majority of their patients have complaints stemming from stress associated with problems in living rather than from organic disease. In addition, common threads run through these complaints: chronic low self-esteem; alienation from self, especially in the area of sexuality; and alienation from others in the area of intimacy, due primarily to a lack of basic human communication skills. Marriage breakdown, a common outcome of these kinds of alienation, often contributes to considerable illness behavior.

Many, if not most, people tend to avoid confronting and trying to solve the problems of living, preferring instead to seek instant remedies to ameliorate the accompanying distress or pain, be these remedies pharmacological or religious. Valium®, for example, has made more money for its manufacturers than any other drug in the entire pharmacopoeia. Suicidal behavior is rampant, especially among the young and the isolated; violence and anomie are widespread. Psychiatrists have long waiting lists and the beds of psychiatric hospitals are always full.

These maladaptive behaviors are hardly a recent phenomenon. The traditional solution to these problems has been an appeal, in our Christian society, to turn to Jesus Christ. While Christian apologists continue to claim that there is not enough religion in the lives of people, the humanist view is that it is time to entertain the contrary hypothesis: that religious socialization contributes to human illness. In 1958, Nathan Ackerman, the founder of family therapy, stated the problem this way: "We are not yet finding our way to the sources of contamination in human relations so as to build immunity against illness and promote positive mental health."[8] Taking a fresh look at some of the root causes of many human ills, we contend that they may in fact lie in the deeply indoctrinated notions of the Christian church acting on men and women, generation after generation. One simple illustration of this connection between religious indoctrination and illness is the relationship between Christian attitudes about anger and peptic ulcers. Investigations into the causes of this condition have revealed quite conclusively that an inability to express anger in a healthy adaptive manner is one of the factors directly contributing to the development of ulcers. For centuries, Christianity has taught that anger is one of the seven deadly sins, an attitude that has been driven deeply into Western child-rearing practices, thus making it difficult for a child to learn healthy approaches to this normal human emotion.

To suggest that Christian teachings may be harmful to human beings puts one in the same precarious position as the first researchers who dared to say that cigarette smoking was harmful to one's health. After all, they were sullying a tradition of adult behavior as well as challenging the very powerful tobacco companies.

When we examine the impact of cigarette smoking on health, we can ask the question in two ways: How does smoking produce the damage? And why do some people escape being damaged by cigarette smoke while others end up with lung cancer? We must question the effects of Christian doctrine in the same way. Why do some people apparently escape being harmed by that doctrine while others seem to be severely traumatized? While we need to pose this question in our dealing with the noxious impact of Christian doctrine, we are no closer to a full answer than those examining the connection between smoking and rates of lung cancer.

We have a partial answer, however, if we fall back on an analogy with communicable diseases. During an epidemic of measles or chickenpox, not everyone exposed to the virus becomes ill; the immune system of some people protects them from the disease. Others' immune systems fail to protect them. In the case of the toxicity from religious indoctrination, an individual's innate humanism constitutes the immune system. This latent humanism includes the ability to remain skeptical about all things supernatural; to like oneself even in the face of Christianity's promotion of self-hate; to experience pleasure, including sexual pleasure, in a responsible way without too much guilt; to form healthy human-to-human bonds in contrast to Christianity's emphasis on the human-to-god bond; and to be tolerant of such dysphoric affects as anger, in spite of Christianity's attempt to promote guilt in the presence of such feelings. Such "innate humanists" may still call themselves Christians, but, luckily for them, the messages do not really "take." The doctrine fails to penetrate to the point where it affects their attitudes and behavior to any great extent. We cannot know how apparently healthy Christians would experience life had they not been so indoctrinated. Nor can we gauge how truly "happy" the TV born-again Christians really are, any more than we know how "happy" the manic-depressive is during a manic phase.

Returning to cigarette smoking, we may offer another parallel between this behavior and the hazards of Christian teachings. Researchers are now convinced that people do not have to be smokers themselves to be harmed by the smoke exhaled by nicotine addicts; second-hand smoke may be every bit as noxious. The same thing is true of Christian teachings. For one thing, it is impossible to escape exposure to testimonials, at times ad nauseam, from believers about the wonders of being "saved," "finding Jesus," "living in Christ," "doing God's work," and so on. The doctrines and teachings of the Christian church have permeated our society extensively and penetrated it deeply, affecting our attitudes about every aspect of our lives, often without our realizing it. In the United States, the existing constitutional guarantee of separation between church and state appears to provide little actual "freedom from religion" for the average citizen. In Canada, there is no such constitutional separation, and most legislators come from Christian backgrounds. In Ontario, the legislature forced the Speaker to back down on his plan to abolish the Lord's Prayer from the opening of the legislature. In both Canada and the United States, educational institutions are dominated by Christians committed to proselytization in one form or another.

The Christian religion is a complex subject, an examination of which will take place in subsequent chapters. To introduce the subject, it helps to speak of doctrinal religions and mystical religions. In religions, such as Christianity, that are mainly doctrinal, adherents are encouraged to believe what the church teaches them, and to live their lives in accordance with those beliefs as well as to practice the prescribed rituals. Paul, in his second letter to the Thessalonians, warns his readers, "And we have confidence in the Lord touching you, that ye both do and will do the things which we command you."

In mystical religions the individual is encouraged to find his or her own way to a spiritual oneness with the universe, chiefly through various forms of meditation. Predominantly doctrinal religions such as Christianity have had their share of mystics, some of whom figure prominently in the history of the church. But as the church became more powerful, more bureaucratic, and more allied with the secular power, it became less tolerant of the mystics in its midst to the point where it now discourages people from experiencing God in any direct mystical way. The present multiplicity of denominations within the Christian church (with 74 distinct denominations in the yellow pages of the Toronto phone directory alone) stems largely from conflicts between doctrine and the "direct experience" of "God."

This divisiveness within the church, however, does not prevent believers of all stripes from viewing themselves as the sole importers into human experience of the two great M's, Meaning and Morality. Indeed, Christian clerics have a habit of using the word "moral" as a synonym for "religious," the implication being that one cannot be moral if one is not religious and, conversely, that a religious person cannot possibly be immoral, in spite of a mountain of evidence to the contrary. But as Charles Watts pointed out early in this century, "Whatever value religion may possess, it has no necessary connection with morality. The two were distinct in their origin, they may have been disassociated in their history, and they still exist apart from each other. The Rationalist is impressed with the fact that it is morality that has modified religion, not religion that has modified morality."[9] We shall return to this point in chapter 11.

There is in fact, no evidence that religious socialization or "being religious" promotes moral behavior. Indeed, the opposite case can be made, namely, that indoctrination with Christian god-talk is incompatible with the psychological growth required for moral development of human beings. This view holds that those believers who do lead moral lives do so *in spite of,* and not because of, their religious socialization and beliefs.[10]

A common charge leveled at behavioral scientists by religionists is that they function in a framework essentially devoid of considerations of morality and meaning. And this criticism is valid. Behavioral scientists have been most reluctant to extend their conceptual models to include a consideration of values and ethics for the simple reason that this would logically lead to a belief system that was uncompromisingly humanistic, thereby stepping on religionists' toes. One example is provided by psychoanalytic ego psychology, which is concerned with the issue of adaptation, a term referring to an individual's coping ability, or the power to master each successive stage in bio-psycho-sexual development in all its dimensions—internal, interpersonal, and environmental. In simpler terms, it has to do with problem-solving capacity; the word "competence" is used to designate how well an individual solves the problems associated with each of these life stages.

When faced with the existential issues of mortality, suffering, and the mysteries of the unknown, a truly competent individual has no need to fall back on prepackaged Christian solutions to these existential problems, since this would compromise the competence he or she has developed to solve other problems. If a person's interpersonal competence is sound, he or she should be able to develop the human support systems to help cope with the angst we all feel when confronted with human suffering as well as the unexplained and the inexplicable. Such a truly competent person would have no need for a set of externally imposed rules governing sexual and social behavior. He or she would naturally learn that individuals can thrive only where each is concerned with the well-being of the human group that provides them with support; and such an awareness would be more likely to produce moral behavior than where rules of moral behavior are divinely inspired and imposed from above.

It is not too extreme to suggest that behavioral scientists, in order to avoid conflict with the religionist establishment, have made an "unconscious" political decision not to concern themselves with the logical values implications of their theoretical constructs. But those who claim a scientific orientation to their work would be wise to heed the words of John McKinnon Robertson who pointed out, "A man who is either hazy or orthodox on these religious matters is so far ill-prepared to think rightly on any other subject."[11]

As a result of this cautious attitude toward ethical implications of their theoretical apporoaches, health clinicians often function like boxers wearing straitjackets. They pretend that they are concerned only with health and not with ethical belief systems, whereas in reality, most of the interventions they make are value-laden. The simple task of trying to help patients come to terms with their suppressed or repressed anger toward their parents carries with it the value message that it is all right to be angry at one's parents, thus flying directly in the face of the Judeo-Christian command to "honor thy father and thy mother," not to mention the injunction against the "deadly" sin of anger. Self-pleasuring (masturbation), a practice still considered a sin by the Roman Catholic church, is often used as part of the treatment in helping patients overcome sexual problems.

There are other ramifications to this struggle to avoid the issue of values. All the psychological conceptual models we possess in the mental health field (psychoanalysis, ego psychology, learning theory, systems theory, and so on), rich as many of them are in explanatory power, have limitations to their comprehensiveness. They are, after all, explanatory models and not ideologies. Freud was fond of quoting the French physician and neurologist J. M. Charcot, who said, "Theory is good but it doesn't prevent things from existing."[12]

Curious, thinking clinicians in the field, coming face to face with the limitations of existing psychological theories, are confronted with a fork in the road, which requires them to move in a new direction and search for greater understanding both of human behavior and the origins of human suffering. One of these routes is the biological, the other the social. Many inducements beckon researchers in the biological direction. The questions are easier to pose; in the social realm it is difficult to know which questions to ask. In addition, most of the social questions carry political implications not present in most areas of biological research. The researcher looking for answers among genes, neurons, or polypeptides is not likely to get into political hot water. However, the scientist trying to examine the role played by Christian approaches to sexuality in the promotion of rape and child sexual molestation would likely have a struggle to get funding for such a study, even if a satisfactory research methodology were available. Biological research is supported in many ways by the vast biomedical pharmaceutical industrial complex with its vested interest in the increasing medicalization of suffering. Most of those concerned with what society is doing to people are members of the so-called protest groups that lack financial resources to do more than stay alive, let alone fund research projects.

Even more indicative of the phobic attitude of mental health professionals toward the issue of religious socialization is the almost universal avoidance of the topic of god-talk when assessing a patient with a psychiatric problem. As Paul Pruyser has pointed out, the taboo on the part of mental health workers against discussing religion may be more profound than that surrounding the discussion of sex.[13] Psychiatric residents, for example, often present case reports of individuals, couples, and families, which are very comprehensive and well formulated in terms of psychodynamics, biology, or systems concepts. Often these same case histories contain multitudinous references to the patient's religious background, such as "the father came from a rigid Irish Catholic background," "mother's father has a Presbyterian minister," and so on. But the possibility that the patient's experiences with religion could have had some role to play in the production of symptoms is never entertained. Much of this avoidance is related to internal conflict in those clinicians who are either still believers themselves, or closet humanists not yet ready to exorcise the religionist demons of their childhood by using the scientific knowledge and human understanding they have acquired in their professional lives.

Before we can demonstrate how Christian doctrine contributes to ill health, we must first of all be clear about what we mean by the word "health." As the World Health Organization definition asserts, health should ideally be considered as a state of complete physical, mental, and social well-being and not merely the absence of disease. Two things stand out about this definition, one being the emphasis on the positive aspect of health rather than the negative, and the other being the unified nature of this state. The division of the human being into "body" and "mind" has many drawbacks to it, not the least of which is that evocation of a more archaic and, as we shall see, destructive, dichotomy of "flesh" and "spirit."

It seems more useful to postulate that human beings function in at least six interrelated modes: perceptual, cognitive, affective, biological, behavioral, and verbal. When events occurring in any of these six modes are in harmony with events occurring in the others, functioning is optimal. Under these circumstances individuals are likely to speak their thoughts freely; express their feelings relatively openly; and behave in accordance with their feelings, attitudes, and beliefs. Their autonomic nervous systems are likely to function in a smooth and integrated fashion with all the other modes. People in this state may be regarded as healthy, emanating a kind of wholeness and integrity.[14] Living in harmony with their own human impulses and reactions, they are more likely to live in harmony with others than those who, under the influence of Christianity, are socialized to live in a constant state of war with themselves. As this book will demonstrate, development along "healthy" lines is more likely to occur in a humanistic environment, uncontaminated by the kind of messages inherent in Christian indoctrination.

The behavioral sciences have much to tell us about those patterns of child rearing that tend to produce mental health or ill health. The prevalent view in the nineteenth century was that children were miniature adults to be seen but not heard; whose heads were empty vessels to be filled with aphorisms, often of a religious nature; and whose willfulness had to be curbed by liberal applications of the rod. By contrast, children are now thought to arrive in this world with a collection of innate potentialities, the unfolding of which depends largely on interaction with caretaking and caring adults. The development (or stunting) of these potentialities takes place around such issues as the gratification and frustration of biological needs; the fulfillment of affectional needs through both verbal and tactile means; and the child is taught to cope with his or her sexuality as well as with such dysphoric affects as anger, disappointment, and sadness. Modern theories of child rearing also assess the manner in which caring adults foster or frustrate children's attempts to master their own environment—external, internal, and inter-personal—as they move from clumsiness to competence in the process. Finally, they include the issue of behavioral controls.

Before moving on to define religion and to examine Christian doctrine specifically, it is necessary to emphasize one point. Throughout this book we are concerned about the impact of Christian doctrine on individuals in our society, as that doctrine acts through the family, the educational systems, and the churches themselves. Generally we are not very concerned with the phenomenon of "being religious." This is a crucial distinction. It is possible for the early life of an individual to be markedly influenced by caretakers who transmit a number of doctrinal messages, whether or not they see themselves as being Christian. Such an individual may never view himself or herself as religious at all, but still live a life that has been profoundly shaped by Christian doctrine. The doctrinal messages of Christianity are woven into the fabric of the society and, while these messages are more likely to be reinforced in those people who go to church, they also act on people who do not. In many instances the doctrinal messages are encoded in secular legislation such as those laws regarding sexuality and reproduction.

Some would argue that mine are merely theoretical assumptions derived from clinical experience, and in that sense they are correct. The views expressed here have not been subjected to rigorous scientific examination; and certainly they should be tested as rigorously as research methodology will allow. But there lies the rub. The methodology for testing these hypotheses is a long way from being developed; indeed, the design appropriate for studying this question may never be developed.

But however valuable rigorous research studies are, counting and measuring is not the only scientific tool at the disposal of human reason—except in the case of those scientists for whom mathematical-type proof is the new religious dogma. Erich Fromm, in discussing the role of academic psychology in understanding religion, put it this way: "It was more often concerned with insignificant problems which fitted an alleged scientific method than with devising new methods to study the significant problems of man."[15] We humans desperately need new ways of conceptualizing our problems, so that we can stop using "solutions" that make these problems worse.

One of these "solutions" continues to be Christian doctrine.

NOTES

1. Jules Henry, *Pathways to Madness* (London: Jonathan Cape, 1972), p. 66.

2. Karen Armstrong, *The Gospel According to Woman* (London: Elm Tree Books, 1986), p. ix.

3. David Mechanic, "Illness Behavior, Social Adaptation and the Management of Illness," *The Journal of Nervous and Mental Disease* 165, no 2. (August 1977): 79.

4. Ibid.

5. Norman F. White. "Can Faith Heal?" *Canadian Family Physician* 30 (January 1984): 125–29.

6. James Randi, *The Faith Healers* (Buffalo, N.Y.: Prometheus Books, 1989).

7. Charles Y. Glock and Rodney Stark, *Religion and Society in Tension* (Chicago: Rand McNally & Company, 1965), p. 290.

8. Nathan W. Ackerman, *The Psychodynamics of Family Life* (New York: Basic Books Inc., 1958), p. 343.

9. Charles Watt. "The Meaning of Rationalism," in Gordon Stein, ed., *An Anthology of Atheism and Rationalism* (Buffalo, N.Y.: Prometheus Books, 1980), p. 24.

10. Wendell W. Watters, "Moral Education: Homo Sapiens or Homo Religiosus?" in Paul Kurtz, ed., *Building a World Community* (Buffalo, N.Y.: Prometheus Books, 1989), pp. 283–90.

11. John Mackinnon Robertson. "Godism," in *An Anthology of Atheism and Rationalism,* p. 70.

12. In James Strachey, trans. and ed., *The Complete Psychological Works of Sigmund Freud* (London: The Hogarth Press, 1962), 3: 13n.

13. Paul W. Pruyser. "An Assessment of Patient's Religious Attitudes in the Psychiatric Case Study," *Bulletin of the Menninger Clinic* 35 (1971): 272–91.

14. W. W. Watters, M.D., A. Bellissimo, Ph.D., and J. S. Rubenstein, M.D., "Teaching Individual Psychotherapy: Learning Objectives in Communication," *Canadian Journal of Psychiatry* 27, no. 4 (June 1982): 263–69.

15. Erich Fromm, *Psychoanalysis and Religion* (New Haven, Conn.: Yale University Press, 1974), p. 6.

2

Christianity: Its Doctrine and Strategies

"But foolish and unlearned questions avoid, knowing that they do gender strifes."

—2 Tim. 2:23

"All the creeds were made by men, and men only, and for the most part by men whose names even we do not know, and who certainly had no more authority to impose their views on the world than you or I would have."

—Alfred Henry Tyrer (1936)[1]

Intellectual life in the Western world has been dominated by Christianity for centuries. An unquestioning attitude regarding religion still prevails throughout much of society; for example, in very few public schools do we find a full, open exploration of the role of religion in human history. Part of this failure to examine religion critically is inherent in its very nature, faith being "the substance of things hoped for, the evidence of things not seen" (Heb. 11:1). But much of the pressure to accept Christianity uncritically comes from the church itself; a mere three centuries ago, death could be the punishment for asking "foolish and unlearned questions." We should be thankful that we can now ask the question "What is religion?" without risking the rack or fearing the flames.

In 1910, psychologist William James described religion as "the feelings, acts, and experiences of individual men in their solitude, so far as they apprehend themselves to stand in relation to whatever they may consider the divine."[2] James, operating from the perspective of individual psychology, was not

25

interested in religion as a social institution. Sociologist Émile Durkheim stated in 1915: "A religion is a unified system of beliefs and practices relative to sacred things, that is to say things set apart and forbidden—beliefs and practices which unite into one single community called a Church, all those who adhere to them."[3] In 1965, Charles Glock and Rodney Stark synthesized a number of more recent sociological perspectives in this definition: "Religion or what societies hold to be sacred, comprises an institutionalized system of symbols, beliefs, values, and practices focused on questions of ultimate meaning."[4]

In 1950, Erich Fromm defined religion as "any system of thought and action shared by a group which gives the individual a frame of orientation and an object of devotion."[5] C. D. Batson and W. L. Ventis, writing from a sociopsychological perspective in 1982, defined religion as "whatever we as individuals do to come to grips personally with questions that confront us because we are aware that we and others like us are alive and that we will die. Such questions we shall call existential questions."[6]

These definitions, appearing as they do over a period of some eighty years, tell us a great deal about the change in the academic approach to the study of religion. Both James and Durkheim, in the early part of the century, made the "divine" and the "sacred" central to their frame of reference, as if meaning *had to* be viewed in absolutist terms and from a theistic perspective. Glock and Stark make it clear that religion is only one approach to dealing with questions of ultimate meaning. The definition of Batson and Ventis is on the opposite end of the spectrum from that of James and Durkheim, in that they make the human quest for answers to existential questions the central issue and do not even mention the supernatural.

A comprehensive definition was formulated by S. H. Alatas in 1977.[7] Religion is characterized by seven traits: (1) belief in a supernatural being or beings and belief that man will establish a personal relationship with that being or beings; (2) certain rights and beliefs sanctioned by that supernatural reality; (3) the division of life into sacred and profane; (4) belief that the supernatural communicates its will through human messengers; (5) the attempt to order life in harmony with the truth according to supernatural designs; (6) the belief that the revealed truth supercedes other types resulting from human efforts; and (7) the practice of creating a community of believers. Taking into account that "any definition of religion is likely to be satisfactory only to its author,"[8] "religion" for our purposes is *that system of beliefs that looks to divine supernatural forces for the meaning of human existence and for the rules of behavior designed to cope with existential anxieties.*

Defining the entity "religion" is one thing; examining ways of being religious gets us closer to the experience of the individual. A number of attempts have been made to examine what it means to "be religious."

Glock and Stark have identified five dimensions of religion: the experiential, the ideological, the ritualistic, the intellectual, and the consequential. In their own words:

> The experiential dimension gives recognition to the fact that all religions have certain expectations however imprecisely they may be stated, that the religious person will at one time or another achieve direct knowledge of ultimate reality and will experience religious emotion.
> The ideological dimension is constituted . . . by expectations that the religious person will hold to certain beliefs.
> The ritualistic dimension encompasses the specifically religious practices expected of religious adherence.
> The intellectual dimension has to do with the expectation that the religious person will be informed and knowledgeable about the basic tenets of his faith and its sacred scriptures.
> The consequential dimension . . . is different in kind from the first four. It encompasses the secular effects of religious belief, practice, experience, and knowledge on the individual . . . the consequential dimension deals with man's relation to man rather than with man's relation to God."[9]

It is the consequential dimension of the Christian religion that concerns us here: What is the likely or potential impact on the average citizen (whether or not he or she is currently a believer) of some sixteen centuries of Christianity in its experiential, ideological, ritualistic, and intellectual dimensions?

In 1967, G. W. Allport and J. M. Ross[10] developed a way of categorizing being religious that has continued to have a high profile in the field of the psychology of religion. To them, "intrinsically" religious people were those in whom the faith was an end in itself, whereas "extrinsically" religious people were those who viewed their religion as a means to certain ends. Extrinsically religious people *used* their religion, while intrinsically religious people *lived* theirs. These investigators also developed scales for measuring intrinsic and extrinsic motivation. Since these concepts were developed with American Christians in mind, it's worth examining them in the context of Christian doctrine to see if they are theoretically sound.

The extrinsically religious person is one who presumably attends church because of the social and political advantages, whereas the intrinsically religious person is preoccupied with more internal events having to do with spiritual matters, their relation to God in Christ and the hope of salvation, or joy in being already "saved." When one realizes that the most powerful incentive for people to embrace Christianity was the promise of eternal bliss in the arms of Jesus, coupled with the threat of eternal damnation if they rejected Christianity, it is very difficult to talk about an intrinsic motivation at all. Both types of religious people indulge in religious behavior for what they hope to get out of it. The expected rewards for the "extrinsically" religious are short-term social ones; in the case of the so-called intrinsically religious, the individual's rewards are long-term ones.

In 1982, Batson and Ventis published a review of the social psychological research literature on the impact of being religious, Glock and Stark's consequential dimension. However, they added a third category of being reliqious to the Allport and Ross categories of extrinsic and intrinsic. This third orientation, which they call "religion as a quest," is defined as "an approach that involves honestly facing existential questions in all their complexities, while resisting clear-cut, pat answers."[11] The differences between the quest orientation on the one hand and the intrinsic and extrinsic orientations on the other, are so great that to subsume them all under the rubric "religion" makes no sense whatever. Anyone who resists "clear-cut answers" could hardly be called religious by most definitions of the word, since it is the appeal of such answers that draws people into the god-talking fold. Atheistic secular humanists are preoccupied with existential questions and the issues of morality and meaning, but in no way can their behavior be considered religious; it is in fact the antithesis of traditional religious behavior.

Others blur this crucial distinction between humanism and religion. Erich Fromm uses the oxymoron "humanistic religions" to contrast with authoritarian religions. In his book *Psychoanalysis and Religion,* Fromm states: "One aspect of religious experience is the wondering, the marvelling, the becoming aware of life and of one's own existence, and of the puzzling problem of one's relatedness to the world."[12] This use of the word "religious" to apply to such a truly human activity demonstrates the degree to which god-talk has penetrated human consciousness. Such questioning and wondering often leads individuals to accept religious answers to their questions, which is not surprising given the fact that our religiously dominated educational systems do not encourage humanistically oriented strategies for helping young people to deal with unanswerable existential questions. Freud made the same point in *The Future of an Illusion:* "Critics persist in describing as 'deeply religious' anyone who admits to a sense of man's insignificance or impotence in the face of the universe, although what constitutes the essence of the religious attitude is not this feeling but only the next step after it, the reaction to it which seeks a remedy for it."[13]

In most religions, the great unknown and unknowable is conceptualized as a supernatural, divine, all-powerful being. In the Christian version this entity has been anthropomorphized into a male whose depiction in the Scriptures runs the gamut from vicious and punitive to loving and forgiving, but whose main characteristics seem to be an all-consuming narcissism and a frightening capriciousness. Many theistic religionists who reject the traditional Christian interpretation of God view the deity as a vague spirit or life force that is ubiquitous. Fromm puts it this way: "God is a symbol of man's own powers which he tries to realize in his own life, and is not a symbol of force and domination, having power over man."[14] Fromm's view of God is the antithesis of the Christian view as expressed by Thomas à Kempis in his book *The Imitation of Christ,* which is often reputed to be "the best loved, most widely read religious book in the world after the Bible."[15] Thomas states: "He that hath true and perfect love attributeth nothing that is good to any man, but wholly refereth it unto God, from whom as from a fountain all things proceed; in whom finally all the saints do rest as in their highest fruition."[16] Fromm's view of God is, therefore, clearly heretical to the Christian in light of the following injunction: "Thou oughest therefore ascribe nothing of good to thyself, nor do thou attribute virtue unto any man; but give all onto God without whom man hath nothing."[17]

Fromm's view of God is also the one propounded by Ludwig Feuerbach, a nineteenth-century German philosopher who postulated that religion was essentially an objectification and projection of the most noble of subjectively experienced human attributes, particularly those having to do with loving, willing, and thinking. For Feuerbach there was or should be no distinction between the human and the divine, the subjective and the objective. As he put it, "the object of any subject is nothing else than the subject's own nature taken objectively."[18] Feuerbach added, "for the qualities of God are nothing else than the essential qualities of man himself."[19] He elucidates this process further: "Man—and this is the mystery of religion—projects his being into objectivity and then again makes himself an object of this projected image of himself thus converted into a subject; he thinks of himself not as an object of himself, but as the object of an object, of another being than himself."[20] Feuerbach viewed Christianity as an example of extreme objectification of a particularly destructive sort in that it was the best human attributes that were projected onto the objectified god, whereas the most undesirable human attributes remained with the human being in the form of original sin. God became the source of love and God's will became the issue rather than man's ability to love, to will, and to think. Feuerbach once claimed that his principal aim was to change "the friends of God into friends of man, believers into thinkers, worshipers into workers, candidates for the other world into students of this world, Christians who on their own confession are half animal and half angel into men—whole men."[21]

This view of God is essentially that of secular humanism with god-talk added. If human beings could take back all the good parts of themselves that have heretofore been projected onto the image of God, the concept of divinity would become empty, a fossilized record of the cultural history of the human race.

In his book *Christ and Freud,* Arthur Guirdham dismisses, along with Fromm, the Christian God. But for Guirdham, the Eastern mystical religions hold the key to understanding the deity; to know "God," the individual must totally abandon "self." Guirdham sees the individual human being as a "dimly apprehended instrument of a more universal influence rather than as a separately functioning personality."[22] For Fromm, the religious person should be concerned with developing his or her human potential to the fullest; for Guirdham, being religious involves literally the opposite process, trying to lose the self in a contemplation of the infinite.

We are then left with two commonly accepted versions of God, the Christian, authoritarian, anthropomorphized male version and the more eastern mystical version. Many religious people hold to a vague amalgam of these two views.

The mystical religious approach to God relies heavily on direct experiencing of God through the act of meditation, a losing of self in an attempt to effect a union with the infinite. Guirdham points out that the true mystic is "less than all others susceptible to human influences."[23] This statement is a bald indictment of religion and of its influence in human society. Why would people need to put themselves into a state beyond human influences if it weren't for the belief that human influence was painful or evil? Unfortunately, as we will see in subsequent chapters, religious solutions to the painfulness of human interaction in the past have led to beliefs and practices that make human interaction ever more painful. Any mental health clinician who works with couples and families knows that the emotional withdrawal of one member of the family, whether it be accompanied by prayer, bible reading, sulking in one's room, a trip to the corner tavern, or a schizophrenic episode, is incompatible with adaptive functioning in that family.

ORIGINS OF THE CHRISTIAN CHURCH

The real Jesus, "whose name is not so much written as ploughed into the history of this world,"[24] still refuses to stand up, having never emerged from behind more than a hundred years of scholarship devoted to the quest. Theories regarding Jesus range from the view that if such a person ever existed, he saw himself as the Messiah of the Jews and carefully and skillfully manipulated events to conform to ancient prophecies,[25] to the idea that he was a humanistically oriented rabbi who was exceptionally intuitive and perceptive about human behavior.[26] One major task of scholarly work in this area has been to determine what Jesus actually said during his brief career (as a teacher, a preacher, or a politician, depending on one's views), since practically everything written about him was set down by people who had very definite views regarding his status in the universe. Whoever and whatever Jesus was, it hardly seems fair to make him responsible for the institution that grew up in his name to become the predominant religion of the Roman Empire less than four centuries after his death and to go on to be the largest religion, numerically, on earth today. Emerson's definition of an institution as "the lengthened shadow of one man"[27] does not really fit the case of Jesus and the Christian church.

During the fifty years following the death of Jesus on the cross nothing was written down, primarily because his followers expected his imminent return to Earth. Edward Gibbon captured the mood of early Christianity with these words: "The ancient Christians were animated by a contempt for their present existence, and by a just confidence of immortality, of which the doubtful and imperfect faith of modern ages cannot give us any adequate notion."[28]

When it finally dawned on the faithful flock that Jesus' return to Earth would be delayed indefinitely, they faced the task of building a terrestrial home in order to keep the faith alive. It was at this point, long after Paul had started composing his letters to the struggling churches throughout Asia Minor, that Christians began writing down the oral tradition concerning the events of Jesus' life and teachings. At the earliest, this process began after the fall of Jerusalem in 70 A.D.

I am reminded here of a parlor game I used to play as a boy. All the players sit in a circle. One person begins by whispering a short story to the person on his or her left, and each player repeats this process until the circle is completed. The fun of the game is to compare the original with the version that was gradually embellished by being passed through a dozen or so individuals. In spite of the fact that the stories are neutral, in that no one has a vested interest in introducing any bias, they all suffer considerably in the repetitive retelling. As for the facts of Jesus' life, it would be a real miracle if anything of the real truth survived the process of being filtered through thousands of committed believers over a period of almost half a century.

It is truly a remarkable example of human gullibility that the entire edifice of the Christian church rests on such skimpy documentary evidence. The gospels themselves are full of contradictions concerning Jesus' baptism, his early life, and his teachings, as well as the circumstances of his death and supposed resurrection. The gospels we now possess derive from fourth-century collections culled from a wider assortment of versions of Jesus' life and teachings. None of the original manuscripts of the New Testament has survived nor have any direct copies. Biblical scholar R. Joseph Hoffmann puts the situation this way: "What we possess are copies of copies so far removed from anything that might be called a 'primary' account that it is useless to speculate about what an original version of the gospel would have included."[29] Along the way, each new transcription and each new translation was open to alterations, additions, and deletions in accordance with the theological biases of the scribe or translator, or those of his ecclesiastical superiors.

The new religion, moving away from its Jewish roots under the influence of Saul the Hellenized Jew turned Paul the Christian, gradually permeated the entire Roman Empire. By the second century A.D., Christians had attracted the notice of a number of pagan writers. Celsus likened them to "frogs holding a symposium round a swamp, debating which of them is the most sinful." The second-century Greek writer Lucian makes us aware of the fact that the modern cult leaders and TV evangelists are not a new phenomenon when he writes, "So if any charlatan or trickster comes among them, he quickly acquires wealth by imposing on these simple folk."[30]

THE CREED AND ITS STRATEGIES

In spite of the many schisms that have rocked the Christian church throughout its history, there is, surprisingly, a modicum of agreement among modern denominations in regard to the essential points of core doctrine. The creation of that doctrine out of the primitive Christology of Paul and the early Christians was no easy matter; it was literally forged in a series of often bitter and bloody battles with a number of "heresies" that grew up within the church during the first few centuries of its existence. One Christian writer has put it this way: "As a matter of fact, the church owes a great deal to heretics. For she was led to develop her theology largely through the pressure which they brought to bear upon her; correct formulations were necessary if men were to see the error of the heretical systems."[31] The author neglected to add that threats of banishment or death for not accepting the "correct formulations" could have had a bearing on the outcome of this prolonged ideological warfare.

In essence, all Christians believe the following: There is a supernatural being governing the universe, who exists in anthropormorphic form and (until the feminist movement) male gender, whose name is God. He lives in heaven and is thought to represent the embodiment of all goodness. Also dwelling in heaven are lesser beings called angels. A very, very long time ago one of these angels, Lucifer by name, did something to displease God and, along with some of his friends, was kicked out of heaven and landed in a place called hell. Lucifer (also called Satan or the Devil) is seen as the embodiment of everything evil.

Right from the time of Adam and Eve, the serpent and the apple, we human beings have never pleased God very much. It seems that Lucifer got the better of the fight for our souls to the extent that God, in his omniscience, concluded that we human creatures were born into a state of original sin, "a psychological torture rack of philosophical idiocy."[32] However, being a loving god, he decided to redeem us wretches by having a human son born by a process of parthenogenesis to a Jewish woman named Mary. The son was called Jesus. (The Jews, who still see themselves as the chosen people, nonetheless wish he had chosen another race for this particular miracle.) This loving god arranged for his "only begotten son in whom I am well pleased" to, suffer death on the cross. The sacrifice was carried out to save us human beings from the consequences of our wickedness, namely a one-way trip to hell. According to the Old Testament the usual practice was for human couples sacrificing their first-born son to this "loving" all-powerful deity; it was quite a switch for the deity to sacrifice his son.

Jesus did not remain dead, however, but spent three days in a limbo state, then came back to live in human form for a while before ascending into heaven, where he now sits at the right hand of God, his loving father, who forced him to die such a painful, ignominious death. This is called the resurrection on which the entire edifice of the Christian church is built. God, however, having taken his son away from human beings on earth, left us something called the Holy Ghost as a kind of spiritual guard dog. Now Christians had to believe in this three-in-one God (the Father, the Son, and the Holy Ghost, the so-called Trinity). Although modern Christian denominations have widely divergent notions about how to achieve salvation, the general idea was and is that the reward for believing in the Trinity, following the prescribed rituals, and avoiding sin is that the Christian will, like Christ, not really die at the end of biological existence but go to heaven and be with God and Jesus.

While many modern church-going Christians insist that certain points of doctrine are no longer part of their consciously held belief system, the fact is that the doctrine as a whole is relentlessly promoted in all Christian churches in various forms. It is one thing to say that one's human intelligence now precludes the conscious, cognitive acceptance of a certain item of doctrine (for example, that of Original Sin), but quite another to demonstrate that that particular piece of doctrine has not shaped or is not still shaping one's emotional and behavioral reactions and that of other people.

Essentially all Christians believe in the Apostle's Creed:

> I believe in God the Father Almighty, Maker of heaven and earth:
> And in Jesus Christ his only Son our Lord,
> Who was conceived by the Holy Ghost, Born of the Virgin Mary,
> Suffered under Pontius Pilate, Was crucified, died, and was buried: He descended into hell; The third day he rose again from the dead;
> He ascended into heaven, And sitteth on the right hand of God the Father Almighty;
> From thence he shall come to judge the quick and the dead.
> I believe in the Holy Ghost. The holy Catholic Church; The Communion of Saints; The Forgiveness of sins; The Resurrection of the body, And the Life everlasting. Amen.

Throughout its early centuries, the church had the most difficulty coming to grips with the doctrine of the Trinity, and indeed many of the heresies had to do with the essential nature of the three Gods—the Father, the Son, and the Holy Ghost. Having committed itself to the doctrine, the church had to defend it against all comers. One of the three great creeds of the Christian church, the so-called Creed of Saint Athanasius, represented an attempt to "clarify" the church's position on this aspect of doctrine. Each reader must decide for himself how clarifying it actually is. With apologies for its length, those sections having to do with the Trinity are quoted below:

QUICUMQUE VULT*

3. Now the Catholic Faith is this, / that we worship one God in Trinity, and the Trinity in Unity;

4. Neither confusing the Persons, / nor dividing the Substance.

5. For there is one Person of the Father, another of the Son, / another of the Holy Ghost;

6. But the Godhead of the Father, and of the Son, and of the Holy Ghost is all one, / the glory equal, the majesty co-eternal.

7. Such as the Father is, such is the Son, / and such is the Holy Ghost;

8. The Father uncreated, the Son uncreated, / the Holy Ghost uncreated;

9. The Father infinite, the Son infinite, / the Holy Ghost infinite;

10. The Father eternal, the Son eternal, / the Holy Ghost eternal;

11. And yet there are not three eternals, / but one eternal;

12. As also there are not three uncreated, nor three infinites, / but one infinite, and one uncreated.

13. So likewise the Father is almighty, the Son almighty, / the Holy Ghost almighty;

14. And yet there are not three almighties, / but one almighty.

15. So the Father is God, the Son God, / the Holy Ghost God;

16. And yet there are not three Gods, / but one God.

17. So the Father is Lord, the Son Lord, / the Holy Ghost Lord;

18. And yet there are not three Lords, / but one Lord.

19. For like as we are compelled by the Christian verity / to confess each Person by himself to be both God and Lord;

20. So are we forbidden by the Catholic Religion / to speak of three Gods or three Lords,

21. The Father is made of none, / nor created, nor begotten.

22. The Son is of the Father alone; / not made, nor created, but begotten.

23. The Holy Ghost is of the Father and the Son; / not made, nor created, nor begotten, but proceeding.

---

*from *Common Prayer Book,* Anglican Church of Canada (1962).

24. There is therefore one Father, not three Fathers; one Son, not three Sons; / one Holy Ghost, not three Holy Ghosts.

25. And in this Trinity there is no before or after, / no greater or less;

26. But all three Persons are co-eternal together, / and co-equal.

27. So that in all ways, as is aforesaid, / both the Trinity is to be worshipped in Unity, and the Unity in Trinity.

28. He therefore that would be saved, / let him thus think of the Trinity.

If these lines had been written by a patient in the back ward of a mental hospital, we would all agree that they represent an excellent example of the thought processes of a floridly psychotic obsessional. The doctrine of the Trinity continues to elude rational human comprehension, although these words are faithfully repeated week after week by believers in the pews.

The actual origins of Christianity are shrouded in the mists of time; however, that mist has cleared enough to enable scholars to ascertain that its basic tenets could be found in no fewer than fifteen other so-called mystery religions that preceded Christianity or were concurrent with it. They all had five elements in common: (1) a promise of immortality; (2) savior gods who suffered, died, and rose from the dead; (3) the promise of redemption by the suffering savior, who made this supreme sacrifice in order to guarantee both forgiveness of sins and salvation; (4) rebirth through baptism; and (5) sacramental meals by the worshipers, in the belief that this represented the incorporation of the god himself.[33]

Competition among religions in the Roman world, even after Constantine's "conversion" to Christianity, was particularly keen, both in terms of acquiring new converts and in seeking favor with the ruling emperor. The ultimate triumph and continuing success of the Christian religion was due, more than anything else, to the consummate political skill its early fathers demonstrated in developing the strategies that enabled them to "persuade" people to the faith.

CHRISTIAN STRATEGIES FOR PROMOTING THE FAITH

Proselytization

This was by far the most important strategy. In Matt. 28:16–20, Jesus instructs his disciples, "Go ye therefore, and teach all nations, baptizing them in the name of the Father, and of the Son and of the Holy Ghost; teaching them to observe all things whatsoever I commanded you." Modern biblical scholarship suggests that Jesus may not have seen his mission, whatever it was, as having anything to do with Gentiles; it is more likely that this aggressive proselytization was the work of Paul, and that scriptural "authority" for it was placed in Jesus' mouth many decades after his death.[34] Whatever the facts, the early Church had a frenzied commitment to spreading the good news and winning new converts, a commitment that was foreign to all other religions. As one writer put it, "If it [the church] were to refrain from doing so, it would be abandoning its very self."[35]

For centuries, Christian proselytization was accompanied by a variety of persuasive methods, such as the rack, the sword, and later the rifle. The seeds of such inhuman behavior on the part of the Christian church had been laid by Paul in his second epistle to the Thessalonians, when he wrote: "And to you who are troubled, rest with us, when the Lord Jesus shall be revealed from heaven with his mighty angels. In flaming fire taking vengance on them that know not God, and that obey not the gospel of our Lord Jesus Christ, who shall be punished with everlasting destruction from the presence of the Lord and from the glory of his power" (2 Thess. 1:7–9).

In true Godfather tradition, the early church made people an offer they could not refuse. As the historian Edward Gibbon put it: "It became the most sacred duty of a new convert to diffuse among his friends and relations the inestimable blessing which he had received, and to warn them against a refusal that would be severely punished as a criminal disobedience to the will of a benevolent but all-powerful Deity."[36]

Modern Christianity, being more "civilized," no longer relies on such crude methods as physical torture to win souls for God. Modern instruments of proselytization do not leave visible scars, twisted limbs, or dead bodies; Christianity has discovered more psychological forms of torture and has mastered the use of the mass media for this purpose, with the permission and the blessing of the state.

The stated justification for Christian missionary work is the obligation to share the good news about Jesus Christ coming into the world to save us all from the consequences of our sins. But there may be deeper psychological motivation for this behavior. The essential elements of the Christian doctrine so violate natural human intelligence that, as a way of quieting their disturbing doubts, believers are internally pressured to convince others of the validity of that doctrine. Guirdham makes somewhat the same point when he writes: "When the Inquisition persecuted heretics it did not do so because it knew it was right but because it feared it was wrong. Blessed with inward, felt, nonratiocinative certainties, men do not persecute. . . . Every Christian who ever persecuted a fellow being because the latter did not believe in the immortality of the soul or the divinity of Christ was agreeing with his victim."[37]

Erich Fromm has called Christianity a *folie à millions*,[38] an expansion of a term used in psychiatry, *folie à deux*. This is applied to the phenomenon of shared craziness between two people who live together in a relatively isolated state, tied together hy blood, marriage, friendship, belief systems, or necessity.

One member of the dyad develops delusions, usually of a persecutory nature, and tries to get the other to agree with his perception that the neighbor is transmitting subliminal messages on the television set or that the breweries are poisoning the milk to encourage people to drink beer. The "sane" partner has the choice either of agreeing with the "crazy" one or of challenging the correctness of his perceptions and thus creating conflict in the relationship. Unable to risk the rift that might follow from this latter course of action, the "sane" partner goes "crazy" in order to preserve the relationship intact. When Freud, in *Future of an Illusion,* referred to religion as a neurosis, he may have misdiagnosed it by a country mile; the term psychosis may be closer to the mark.

Most Christians, without a moment's hesitation, would say that they subscribe to the so-called Golden Rule, which admonishes us to "Do unto others as you would have them do unto you." However, in all honesty, Christians cannot subscribe to the Golden Rule and remain Christians. Being in possession of The One True Faith, Christians, with their commitment to proselytization, naturally resist pressure from any other religion to convert to its tenets. Given the track record of Christianity toward people who declined the gift offered them by the sacrifice on the cross, there is not much doubt that Christians would rather fight than switch if pressured to worship any other god.

One often overlooked aspect of proselytization is that it depends on the proselytizer being "one up" on the proselytized, who is usually disadvantaged psychologically, socially, or economically, or else in a state of military sub-jugation. This process never takes place between equals; it is always a case of "get 'em when they're down." The smug missionary gloats when he wins another soul for Christ. The televangelist derives more tangible financial rewards from his predatory raids on the lonely, the poor, the elderly, and the uneducated.

Dualism

Critics of modern health care and health care education trace many problems to the mind-body dichotomy that still dominates medical thinking, in spite of some attempts to develop a more holistic approach. This medical dualism is usually traced philosophically to René Descartes, who taught that the mind and the body were essentially separate entities. In laying the blame for the dehumanization of health care at the door of Descartes, we are ignoring the obvious fact that he was a product of a society highly imbued with the doc-trine of the Christian church. From its beginnings, the church had taught a rigidly dualistic conception of the human being: each man and each woman consisted of a "flesh" and a "spirit," and the two were not only destined never to meet but to be at constant war with each other. It is certain that Descartes, in his philosophical musings, must have been more than a little influenced by the intensity of theological debate raging at the time. Four years after Descartes' birth (in 1596), the Italian philosopher Giordano Bruno was burned at the stake by the Inquisition for teaching that "All reality is one in substance, one in cause, one in origin; and God and this reality are one."[39]

The concept of dualism did not originate with the Christians, but has philosophical roots reaching back to Plato and beyond.[40] However, it is safe to say that the Christian version has had the most profound impact on the lives of human beings in the Western world. As a strategy for achieving military and political power, "divide and conquer" has always enjoyed a high popularity; it has proven equally effective in controlling the lives of individual Christians. In George Bernard Shaw's play *Heartbreak House,* the character Ellie Dunn hits the nail on the head with these lines: "We know now that the soul is the body and the body the soul. They tell us they are different because they want to persuade us that we can keep our souls if we let them make slaves of our bodies."[41]

Under the influence of a belief system that promotes such hostility and distrust between two "parts" of the indivisible whole human being, it requires almost superhuman effort for an individual to develop any sense of unity or wholeness, Without integration of the whole person, there can be no real self, no self-esteem, and no true self-mastery. If one buys into the Christian belief system, such integration becomes impossible, and the individual becomes dependent on the authority of the church. Such a divided person is doomed to a life-long fate of irreconcilable conflict between the potential human being struggling for integration and mastery, and the Christian doomed forever to fragmentation and abject groveling at the feet of the Almighty Father.

OTHER STRATEGIES

Proselytization and the promotion of dualism were not the only strategies used by the early Christians in their struggle for political power. Other strategies were equally effective and equally devastating to the human condition. In gaining and keeping control of its followers, the church actively fostered their infantile dependency and, with the promise of a life after death, their infantile greed; it exploited normal human existential fears, and stimulated and manipulated human guilt and ambivalence. In the area of sexuality and reproduction the early fathers developed a set of teachings that essentially made the female uterus a baby factory for producing an endless supply of Christians, teachings that are still causing untold suffering and which should earn for the church the verdict of guilty for having the most vicious demographic aggressor of all time.

Until Johannes Gutenberg's invention of moveable type in the mid-fifteenth century, the church had to rely on its priests and bishops to spread the word orally to the largely illiterate masses throughout Europe. Once the printing press made it possible for increasing numbers of people to read the Bible themselves, the church relied more and more on literary indoctrination to achieve its goals. The book that turned out to be the most useful for this purpose (next to the Bible itself) was *The Imitation of Christ* by German-born Thomas à Kempis who, as a priest in the Augustinian order, lived most of his ninety-two years in Holland. In 1427, the first manuscript version of *The Imitation* appeared, to be followed by many more; a total of over 700 manuscript versions are known to exist. After Gutenberg's invention made the scribe's role redundant, *The Imitation of Christ* grew to become one of the chief literary tools by which the church was able to weave its doctrine into the fabric of Western society. By the end of the nineteenth century, 600 editions had been printed in Latin, 300 in Italian, 350 in German, and "uncounted editions of this choicest devotional handbook of the middle ages had been made in English."[42] Paul M. Bechtel, who edited the 1984 Moody Classic edition, has this to say in his introduction: "This book, read in the spirit of consecration, has given guidance to generations of Christian believers of every persuasion throughout the world."[43]

For someone with any interest in human health and welfare in this final decade of the twentieth century, *The Imitation of Christ* is a frightening document. In passage after passage, the Christian is encouraged to welcome suffering in this world as a way to please the Lord., The poor pilgrim is encouraged to indulge in a veritable orgy of self-hatred and denigration, and to avoid most strenuously any trace of self-esteem or any attempt at self-actualization. Thomas appears to have had an absolute phobia about people, since in passage after passage he advises his readers to avoid human contact and to abjure the development of a human support system. One entire chapter is devoted to warning devout readers to avoid learning of any sort that does not enhance their faith in God.

God is made the speaker in many passages; he repeatedly makes demands for abject, absolute, unquestioning worship in a manner worthy of the most vicious earthly potentate: "Ask not that which is delightful and profitable to thee, but that which is acceptable to me, and tends to promote my honor."[44] According to Thomas, God's monomaniacal zeal knows no bounds: "I am to be praised in all my saints: I am to be blessed above all things, and to be honored in everyone, whom I have thus gloriously exalted and predestined without any precedent merits of their own."[45]

It is a common mistake to dismiss all this as medieval nonsense that has no meaning as the twentieth century draws to a close. Who cares about the bizarre musings of a reclusive fifteenth-century monk? And yet until well into this century this book was in press somewhere in the world every day of the week; and its ideas are still for many throughout the Western world part of the cultural air they breathe. The editor of the 1984 Moody Press edition closes his introduction with these words: "One rejoices in the knowledge that a new edition will add other readers to the company of those who have found springs of livings water in Thomas à Kempis' ageless little book."[46] We shall later explore in depth the effects of these "springs of living water" on the healthy development of normal human beings; the reader will have his or her own opportunity to decide whether "rejoicing" is in fact an appropriate human response.

Many people born into a strongly religious family submit to that belief system throughout their lives; others undergo the long, tortuous, and painful road from believer to humanist. Others drift slowly and passively away from their cradle faith to become lukewarm Christians or "nothingarians" without fully confronting what the religious indoctrination has done to them as human beings.

Many of these lukewarm Christians who are products of mainline Christianity are eventually seduced into fundamentalism, a process that has been described by Edmund D. Cohen in his book *The Mind of the Bible-Believer*.[47] Although Cohen described this process as it applies to extreme fundamentalist conversion, the seven step-wise devices used by fundamentalist god-talkers lay bare the violence done to human reason and dignity by all forms of Christian indoctrination.

In the first device, "The Benign Attractive Persona of the Bible," all kinds of extravagant claims and promises are made implicitly or explicitly in the manner of the old-fashioned snake oil salesman or the modern TV commercial. As part of the program of Christian mind control, the word love is used frequently; however, as we shall see, the word develops an idiosyncratic meaning once the individual is "inside." In the Christian commercial, promises of forgiveness of sins and life everlasting are added to the promise of love. The term "love bombing" has been applied to this process as it refers to modern cults; Cohen refers to this strategy as a "colossal bait and switch sales pitch."[48] Once the individual is "inside," the sugar coating quickly dissolves, leaving the bitter pill.

The second device, "Discrediting the World," calls for subjects to wean themselves away from those former friends and associates who do not share the same belief. Analogously, in *The Imitation of Christ* we find these words, "Trust not to friends and kindred, neither do thou put off the care of thy soul's welfare til hereafter; for men will sooner forget thee than thou art aware of."[49] However, since god-talkers cannot entirely erase human need for human contact, the phenomenon of Christian "fellowship" is encouraged to make sure that new members rub shoulders with well-indoctrinated fellow Christians. Rituals, such as prayer, hymn singing, and communion, play an important part in encouraging the neophyte to withdraw from previous human supports and focus on God and Christ.

One devastating aspect of this device is the discrediting of the individual's human capacity to reason. On this point Cohen states, "while the Bible does not explicitly say that independent thinking is a cardinal sin—to do so would give the game away—it is the crux of any biblically authentic definition of sin, one incompatible with doing the devotional program."[50] Although the Bible may not have explicitly discouraged the use of human reason, it was obvious by the time of Thomas à Kempis that knowledge was to be mistrusted: "My son, in many things it is thy duty to be ignorant and to esteem thyself as dead upon earth, and as one to whom the whole world is crucified."[51]

The third device, "Logocide," refers the killing of words, or rather, the meaning of words. As the Red Queen stated in *Alice in Wonderland,* words were to mean what she chose them to mean. Christian logocide concentrates on words like life, death, truth, wisdom, and, of course, love, none of which carry the accepted, consensual meaning as they issue out of the mouths of god-talkers. Life and death mean life in Christ or death to Christ, and are simply terms denoting belief or unbelief in the risen Lord. Wisdom has nothing to do with human wisdom but rather refers to the level of commitment to the Christian system of beliefs. With the word love being used so freely in god-talking commercials, it is no wonder that confused, frightened, and friendless people would be attracted to an institution promising love; as they understand or imagine love, it is something they have been deprived of and yearned for all their lives. However, it soon becomes apparent that the human love they seek is not the love of the god-talker; those worthies use the word "love" to refer to an unquestioning obedience to God in return for the promise of everlasting life. In addition to this, the kind of human love originally sought by the initiate, is gradually undermined as being inferior, untrustworthy, not to mention unsatisfying when compared to the love of God. As Cohen states, "Christian love is biblically defined as Holy Spirit-aided self-disclipline in internalizing Christian doctrine and performing the devotional program. As manifested in and by the believer, Christian love has hardly anything to do with passion or affection."[52]

In chapter 1, we defined mental health as that state existing when all levels of an individual being—the perceptual, the cognitive, the affective, the biological, the behavioral, and the verbal—function in a more or less smooth, harmonious, integrated manner. This is akin to what Cohen refers to as integrity, which he defines in this way: "We implicitly think of one who is honest with himself about himself as having integrity."[53] The fourth device consists of a relentless assault on this integrity. Since the entire belief system called Christianity requires the individual to accept that belief on faith and to deny the evidence of human intelligence when this conflicts with the belief system, integrity for the Christian becomes impossible.

Hand in glove with the assault on integrity is the fifth Christian device as named by Cohen, the process of "Dissociation Induction." Once the integrity of the believer is compromised to the point where he or she is "hooked," it becomes necessary for the brain-washing process to be intensified through this process of dissociation. One of the chief elements in this strategy is to make believers live in a perpetual state of fear of what is basically germane to their human nature. All emotions are frowned on except for guilt, which is encouraged as a means of mind control. The normal human emotion of anger is categorized as one of the seven deadly sins; the inevitable guilt makes it impossible for the neophyte to mobilize a healthy human response to such inhuman indoctrination.

Any forbidden feeling leading to more guilt causes further dissociation. As Cohen asserts: "The supposed renewal of the mind so that it thinks only godly thoughts, the fatuous peace and tepid joy of the person exhibiting euphoric calm, the apparent absence of friction with other people, these are side effects of a dissociated state of mind."[54]

At a certain point in the Christian mind-control process, pressure mounts to close that mind off completely from the believer's own human intelligence, in order to protect it from any influence not in keeping with the doctrine (the sixth device named by Cohen: "Bridge Burning"). At this point the believer has moved beyond a mere dissociated state into a psychosis, in which genuine interaction between the individual and reality is impossible since the "real world" is perceived solely in terms of the Christian world view. This explains why it is impossible to carry on a true dialogue about existential issues with a committed Christian, programmed as he or she is to respond to the unbeliever with a bemused tolerance, secure in the "belief" that God has some lofty purpose in closing some minds to "the truth." As Cohen puts it, "The content of the teaching, as well as the form of social relations, is set up so as to dig a psychological moat around the believers."[55]

The bottom line in Christian brain-washing is, of course, fear (Cohen's seventh device: "Holy Terror"), which is used only when the believer is well "inside." This fear is grounded in the punishment awaiting Christians who fail to subjugate their human intelligence and will to the wishes of the god-talkers. Cohen asserts that the authors of the New Testament "deliberately contrived the portentious New Testament statements about horrors in the afterlife to be the worst eventualities of which the mind—or at least the ordinary minds of those who would be rank-and-file believers—could conceive."[56]

At first glance Cohen seems to be describing the stages of conversion to the more right-wing fundamentalist evangelical brand of Christianity, especially the electronic kind, and to the various religious cults that feed on the lost youth as well as those disenchanted with mainline Christianity. It is easy to lose sight of the fact that, in accordance with the core doctrine, the same process goes on in the mainline Christian churches, although usually in a more superficial, less fundamentalist manner. Association with one of the mainline denominations, especially if it is only a nominal, unexamined affiliation, is easier for many people who otherwise like to think of themselves as sophisticated, intelligent, and modern. However, this half-hearted attempt to humanize Christianity on the part of some of the mainline churches is proving to be their undoing. Membership in these denominations is dropping while fundamentalist TV evangelists amass huge fortunes.

The explanation for this is as follows. The core doctrine of the Christian church, coupled with the strategies used over the centuries to gain the power the church now enjoys, is so anti-human that many humanistically oriented denominations and god-talkers have tried to soften the messages to make them more palatable to "educated" congregations. This leads to one of two outcomes. The more secure and intelligent members of such congregations begin questioning, and such questioning may start them down the road toward atheism and possibly humanism. Many tarry at various points along that road. Less secure members of the congregation begin to look for a brand of religion that offers vigorous reinforcement of their flagging faith and more protection from the threat of their own human intelligence. Thus the mainline Christian churches are training millions of people to be the "marks" or "pigeons" for the money-hungry TV evangelists.

Having examined the various strategies by which the church gets people to buy its product, we turn to how the elements of this Christian belief system are antithetical to the development of sound health.

NOTES

1. Alfred Henry Tyrer, *Sex, Marriage and Birth Control* (Toronto: Marriage Welfare Bureau, 1936), p. 227.

2. William James, *The Varieties of Religious Experience* (New York: New American Library, 1958), p. 42.

3. Émile Durkheim, *The Elementary Forms of the Religious Life* (London: George Allen and Unwin Ltd., 1915), p. 47.

4. Charles Y. Glock and Rodney Stark, *Religion and Society in Tension* (Chicago: Rand McNally & Company, 1965), p. 4.

5. Erich Fromm, *Psychoanalysis and Religion* (New Haven, Conn.: Yale University Press, 1974), p. 21.

6. C. Daniel Batson and W. Larry Ventis, *The Religious Experience* (New York: Oxford University Press, 1982), p. 7.

7. Syed Hussein Alatas, "Problems of Defining Religion," *International Social Science Journal* 29, no 2 (1977): 213–34.

8. J. Milton Yinger, "Pluralism, Religion and Secularism," *Journal for the Scientific Study of Religion* 6 (1967): 18.

9. Glock and Stark, *Religion and Society in Tension,* p. 20.

10. G. W. Allport and J. M. Ross. "Personal Religious Orientation and Prejudice," *Journal of Personality and Social Psychology* 5 (1967): 432–33.

11. Batson and Ventis, *The Religious Experience,* p. 149.

12. Fromm, *Psychoanalysis and Religion,* p. 94.

13. Sigmund Freud, *The Future of an Illusion,* in James Strachey, trans. and ed., *The Complete Psychological Works of Sigmund Freud* (London: Hogarth Press), 21: 32.

14. Fromm, *Psychoanalysis and Religion,* p. 37.

15. Paul M. Bechtel in his edition of Thomas à Kempis, *The Imitation of Christ* (Chicago: Moody Press, 1980), p. 15.

16. Ibid. p. 49.

17. Ibid. p. 147.

18. Ludwig Feuerbach, *The Essence of Christianity,* trans. George Eliot (Buffalo, N.Y.: Prometheus Books, 1989), p. 12.

19. Ibid. p. 19.

20. Ibid. p. 30.

21. Quoted by Karl Barth in his introductory essay to Feuerbach, *The Essence of Christianity,* p. xi.

22. Arthur Guirdham, *Christ and Freud* (London: George Allen and Unwin, Ltd., 1961), p. 16.

23. Ibid., p. 39.

24. Ralph Waldo Emerson, *Miscellanies 1868* (abridged), p. 120, quoted in James, *The Varieties of a Religious Experience,* p. 43.

25. Hugh J. Schonfield, *After the Cross* (San Diego, Calif.: A. S. Barnes and Company, Inc., 1981).

26. James Breech, *The Silence of Jesus* (Toronto: Doubleday Canada, Ltd., 1982).

27. Ralph Waldo Emerson, "Self Reliance," in *The Essays of Emerson: Essays and Representative Men* (London: Collins Library of Classics), p. 36.

28. Edward Gibbon, *The Decline and Fall of the Roman Empire* (New York: Dell Publishing Co. Inc., 1972), p. 232.

29. R. Joseph Hoffmann, "The Origins of Christianity," *Free Inquiry* 5, no 2. (Spring 1985): 50.

30. Bamber Gascoigne, *The Christians* (London: Granada Publishing, 1978), p. 9.

31. Alan Richardson, *Creeds in the Making* (Philadelphia: Fortress Press, 1981), p. 31.

32. Charles W. Sutherland, *Disciples of Destruction: The Religious Origins of War and Terrorism* (Buffalo, N.Y.: Prometheus Books, 1987), p. 111.

33. Dan Cover and Dall Whitney, "Another Look at Christianity," *Freethought Today* 7, no. 3. (April 1990): 10.

34. Frances Burke Drohan, *Jesus Who? The Greatest Mystery Never Told* (New York: Philosophical Library, 1985).

35. Hans Conzelmann, *History of Primitive Christianity,* trans. John E. Steely (Nashville, Tenn.: Abingdon Press, 1973), p. 17.

36. Gibbon, *The Decline and Fall of the Roman Empire,* p. 223.

37. Guirdham, *Christ and Freud,* p. 72.

38. Fromm, *Psychoanalysis and Religion,* p. 17.

39. Will Durant, *The Story of Philosophy* (New York: Pocket Books, 1953), p. 150.

40. Vern L. Bullough, *Sexual Variance in Society and History* (Chicago: University of Chicago Press, 1976), pp. 163–64.

41. G. B. Shaw, *Hearbreak House,* Act 2, in *Heartbreak House, Great Catherine, and Playlets of War* (London: Constable and Company, Ltd., 1919), p. 77.

42. Thomas à Kempis, *The Imitation of Christ,* pp. 15–16.

43. Ibid., p. 21.

44. Ibid., p. 237.

45. Ibid., p. 266.

46. Ibid., p. 21.

47. Edmund D. Cohen, *The Mind of the Bible-Believer* (Buffalo, N.Y.: Prometheus Books, 1986).

48. Ibid., p. 171.

49. Thomas à Kempis, *The Imitation of Christ,* p. 74.

50. Cohen, *The Mind of the Bible-Believer,* p. 179.

51. Thomas à Kempis, *The Imitation of Christ,* p. 223.

52. Cohen, *The Mind of the Bible-Believer,* p. 223.

53. Ibid., p. 234.

54. Ibid., p. 261.

55. Ibid., p. 341.

56. Ibid., p. 354.

3

Christianity, the Family, and Self-Esteem

"How can we search out and define those noxious components of family relations that a child sops up and incorporates into his evolving self in the early and vulnerable stages of his development?"
—Nathan W. Ackerman (1961)[1]

"Humble yourselves therefore under the mighty hand of God, that he may exalt you in due time."
—1 Peter 5:6

The family plays powerful roles in human society. In addition to its nurturing and protective functions, the family is the primary agency for carrying out the socialization process by which social norms and values become incorporated into the character structure of the growing child. Indeed, so powerful is the family in human society that many revolutionary political movements have, in their initial stages, attempted to destroy its power to maintain the status quo, by appealing directly to children over the heads of their parents.

Jesus said: "If any man come to me, and hate not his father, and mother, and wife, and children, and brethren, and sisters, yea, and his own life also, he cannot be my disciple" (Luke 14:26). In another gospel, Jesus is quoted as saying: "For I am come to set a man at variance against his father, and the daughter against her mother, and the daughter-in-law against her mother-in-law" (Matt. 10:35). The Hitler youth movement was a major component of Nazi policy, while the early years of the Communist government in the former Soviet Union were marked by an attempt to appeal directly to the young. The present-day religious cults are noted for creating rifts between

47

parents and their adolescent children. However, once a movement achieves its revolutionary goals, as in the case of Christianity and communism, it reverses this position and attempts once more to use the family as an ally in maintaining and extending its power.

The individual, the family, and society impact on each other in a variety of ways. While the family is the most powerful agency in the process of socializing the individual, its role in facilitating an individual's attempts to bring about social change may be minimal to nonexistent. Indeed, many who set out to make changes in society do so in opposition to their families; such people, oriented toward the future, grow beyond their families, whose eyes are more fixed on the past. It is no wonder that the family remains such a source of tension as it strives to meet the needs of society as well as those of its own members who are struggling to achieve their full potential. This is particularly so since such self-actualization sometimes involves individuals in activities designed to make real changes in society and, with these, an altered role for the family.

An ancient Chinese curse goes, "May you live in an era of change." Theoretically, the task of the family would be easier in a society that was stable, in contrast to one in a state of flux. Whether stable, smoothly functioning societies ever existed, except as figures of our nostalgic imagination, is a matter for debate, but certainly ours is not one of them. Indeed, the rate of technological and social change in the developed world places an enormous adaptational burden on the family and on the individual. It would be a mistake, however, to assume that persons growing up in a "stable" society are more mentally healthy than those coming of age in a society racked by turmoil.

In one sense, the process of socialization in the family is a simple one. A popular lesson titled "Children Learn What They Live" describes the process this way:

> If a child lives with criticism, he learns to condemn. If a child lives with hostility, he learns to fight. If a child lives with ridicule, he learns to be shy. If a child lives with shame, he learns to feel guilty. If a child lives with tolerance, he learns to be patient. If a child lives with encouragement, he learns confidence. If a child lives with praise, he learns to appreciate. If a child lives with fairness, he learns justice. If a child lives with security, he learns to have faith. If a child lives with approval, he learns to like himself. If a child lives with acceptance and friendship, he learns to find love in the world.

On another level, the process is very complicated. At times the messages transmitted from parent to child are deliberate strategies, as in the case of the mother who physically beats the child or washes his mouth out with soap for using language of which the parents disapprove. At other times, the messages are subtle but nonetheless effective. If the subject of genitals and sex is never mentioned, the child learns that these are unmentionable topics. If a father stops hugging his son at the age of six but continues to hug the boy's twin sister, a message is communicated about the way men should relate to each other physically.

As for the mental health implications of the socialization process, one critical factor is the amount of ambiguity in the messages parents transmit to their children. If father chuckles when he tells his son that little boys do not hit little girls and makes a habit of coming home drunk and beating the boy's mother, he is giving a very mixed message indeed. The mother who forces her children to go to church but never goes herself is certainly acting in a way that is guaranteed to create conflict in the children. Generally, the more consistency and congruity in the messages transmitted by parents to children, the smoother the process of socialization should be; and the more likely the children will grow up mentally healthy.

Because children are preverbal during the important first years of life, attempts by the parents to regulate their reactions and behavior are likewise often nonverbal; for example, physically removing the child when he starts hitting the family dog. However, such nonverbal behavior on the part of the parent is often accompanied by some reinforcing verbalization, to such an extent that children's first words often consist of their attempts to verbalize the behavioral injunctions and commands they have heard so often from their parents. Thus the process of socialization becomes part and parcel of the development of speech. "Bad" boy, "good" boy, "bad" girl, "good" girl, are often among the first words a child says.

Parents, in interacting with their children, are not involved solely in carrying out the dictates of society; they are also fulfilling parental tasks that are nurturant and supportive, or in the interests of family maintenance and protection. A mother pushing her two-year-old son's hand away from his penis or admonishing her three-year-old daughter not to be so boisterous is performing an act of socialization unrelated to nurturance, family maintenance, or protection. A father who cuddles and comforts a small child with a scraped knee is being nurturant; if he moves a chair across the top of the stairway to keep his crawling child from falling, he is performing a family maintenance task.

However, most interventions of parents with their children are mixed acts of nurturance, family maintenance, and socialization. For example, the father comforting the small child with a scraped knee may add to his soothing words an admonition that little girls shouldn't play so roughly or that little boys should learn not to cry when they are hurt. Thus, while parents are performing the familial functions associated with trying to meet their children's adaptational needs, they are also functioning as agents of a wider society in communicating how people should feel, react, and behave under certain circumstances. As we shall see, when parents are inculcated with notions derived from Christian doctrine, these two sets of goals are not always complementary or even compatible.

CHRISTIAN DOCTRINE AND SELF-ESTEEM

In her book *Current Concepts of Positive Mental Health,*[2] psychologist Marie Jahoda reviewed all current concepts of positive mental health and came up with six clusters of concepts bearing on the issue. These are: (1) the attitudes of an individual toward himself; (2) growth, development, or self-actualization; (3) integration; (4) autonomy; (5) perception of reality; and (6) environmental mastery. Significantly, there are many parallels between Jahoda's list of concepts and my own. The differences are minor but perhaps worth mentioning. In my frame of reference, autonomy and environmental mastery are incorporated in the concept of self-actualization or adaptation, and the concepts of integration and perception of reality are not treated as discrete entities but are rather woven into the other themes. Since the purpose of this book is to examine the issue of positive health in relation to the teachings of the Christian church, I have considered separately a few issues which in Jahoda's work are embedded in the other concepts. These are pleasure and pain, guilt, ambivalence, communication, and sexuality and reproduction.

It is noteworthy that the first factor in both lists has to do with the concept of self. While a number of "self" terms, such as self-acceptance, might have been appropriate to use here, a term with a quantitative connotation such as self-esteem seemed preferable. Self-esteem refers to the value an individual assigns to himself or herself as a person. High self-esteem needs to be differentiated from narcissistic bliss, manic euphoria, and competitive triumph, which are all, in a sense, defensive reactions to low self-esteem. Nor should self-esteem be confused with self-indulgence or smugness. It simply refers to the degree to which one accepts and values oneself, warts and all.

Although psychiatrists and psychologists are noted for disagreeing on just about everything, they do all agree that self-esteem, as understood here, is one cornerstone of sound mental health. People who are considered mentally sound generally have a high level of self-esteem; they feel reasonably competent and secure as people; they generally like themselves, and feel capable of being liked and loved by others. In addition, they are capable of manifesting genuine liking and loving for others. People with high self-esteem are able to be appropriately assertive in trying to have their needs met in a non-manipulative, nondestructive way.

Conversely, the one feature common to all psychiatric patients and many chronically ill patients is low self-esteem.

A well-functioning family contributes to the development of self-esteem in growing children by providing for their basic biological needs and by securing an environment in which they can develop autonomy and actualize their human potential. However, it is difficult to understand how any family can perform this task if it is influenced to any degree by the teachings of the Christian church, since that institution's teachings are uncompromisingly antithetical to the development of self-esteem.

To a large extent, Western society presents a value mosaic, with some of its ethical norms contributing to healthy psychological and emotional growth, while others work in the opposite direction. For each family the question is: Which values does this family "choose" to tolerate and nourish and which ones reject outright? Having "chosen," how does the family promote attitudes and behaviors it considers worthwhile, and discourage those it has rejected?

After working with families of disturbed children, sociologist Jules Henry was moved to conclude that many families merely distill the general pathology of the culture into lethal doses.[3] For the purposes of our argument, whether the family does distill the Christian pathology into lethal doses or acts to neutralize the toxicity of the Christian messages coming from society, depends largely on the degree to which the parents themselves have matured beyond the need for the opiates of Christian doctrine, and have successfully immunized themselves against its noxious side effects.

The Christian negative attitude toward self-esteem, often referred to as pride, has at least some roots in ancient Judaism. The code of Jewish laws states, "Pride is an extremely bad vice, and a person is forbidden to become accustomed to it even to the slightest degree, but he should accustom himself to be humble of spirit, as the sages of blessed memory ordained, 'be exceedingly humble of spirit.' "[4] For the true Christian the situation, however, is much worse. He is called upon to believe in the Doctrine of Original Sin and in Christ's sacrifice for others on the cross, and is expected to try to win favor with God by all manner of verbal breast-beating, fault-finding, and confession of sins.

According to Christian teachings, the self is to be abased, not esteemed. Paul's letters contain many warnings against self-love: "Not that we are sufficient of ourselves to think anything as of ourselves: but our sufficiency is of God" (2 Cor. 3:5). "Let nothing be done through strife or vainglory; but in lowliness of mind let each esteem other better than themselves" (Phil. 2:3). "Put on therefore, as the elect of God, holy and beloved, bowels of mercies, kindness, humbleness of mind, meekness, longsuffering" (Col. 3:12). In his second letter to Timothy, Paul placed "lovers of their own selves" in most unpleasant company with the "covetous, boasters, proud, blasphemers, disobedient to parents, unthankful, unholy" (2 Tim. 3:2).

In Thomas à Kempis's *The Imitation of Christ,* there are at least thirty-seven passages that explicitly warn Christians against thinking well of themselves. Here are a few examples: "It is great wisdom and perfection to esteem ourselves as nothing, and to think always well and highly of others."[5] "Take not pleasure in thy natural gifts, or intelligence, lest thereby thou displease God, to whom belongs all the good whatsoever thou hast by nature."[6] "But if I abase myself, and reduce myself to nothing, and draw back from all self-esteem, and reduce myself to dust, thy grace will be favorable to me, and thy light near unto my heart; and all self-esteem, however little, shall be swallowed up in the valley of my nothingness and perish for ever."[7]

In other passages the venerable monk urges his readers to indulge in a veritable orgy of masochism: "Be fiercely angry against thyself, and suffer no pride to dwell in thee; but show thyself so humble, and so very small, that all may be able to walk over thee, and to tread thee down as the mire of the streets. Vain man, what hast thou to complain of?"[8] "Strike my back and my neck too, that my perversity may be conformed to thy will."[9]

These masochistic messages are not confined to the pages of dusty, medieval tomes; they are repeated week after week in the services of mainline Christian churches. In the Prayer of St. Thomas Aquinas, the penitent exclaims, "I come sick to the doctor of life, unclean to the fountain of mercy, blind to the radiance of eternal light, and poor and needy to the Lord of heaven and earth." In a prayer before confession the believer is called upon to plead, "Dear Jesus, help me to make a good confession, help me to find out my sins, help me to be sorry for them, help me to make up my mind not to sin again." In an Anglican Communion prayer we find these words: "We are not worthy so much as to gather up the crumbs under thy Table."

Abasing and being furiously angry with oneself; labeling oneself as "sick," "unclean," "blind," "poor and needy," and "not worthy to gather crumbs" as a strategy for inveigling favors from a remote divinity, are hardly compatible with the development of healthy self-esteem. Those who allow such messages to penetrate their consciousness to any extent are likely to experience intense conflict between the human being and the believer. As we saw in chapter 1, conflict of this kind is a source of stress, and intense stress constitutes one factor in the production of many illnesses. It is a tribute to the resilience of the species, that any human being could be subjected to this kind of steady indoctrination and yet grow up with any degree of self-acceptance, let alone self-esteem. Brain-washing of this intensity has a powerful impact. The negative self-image thus formed lies at the bottom of many health problems. Furthermore, this tendency to be self-derogatory is transmitted from generation to generation—even in families no longer religious. It finds expression in the behavioral control strategies used in families with small children; phrases such as "bad boy" and "bad girl" are often among the first words used by children, frequently echoing parents who use words like these when they are trying to correct inappropriate conduct. The focus, in true Christian tradition, is on the child's innate badness rather than on the inappropriateness of the behavior. Many parents fail to see the difference between saying to a child, "you are a bad, naughty boy for doing that," and telling the child that a particular mode of behavior is unacceptable and will not be tolerated in the family.

Christians are taught that it is sinful to regard oneself as intrinsically worthy; only God can assign a value to an individual Christian by "saving" him from his sins. By emotionally flagellating themselves and proclaiming their intrinsic worthlessness and emptiness, Christians try to manipulate God into feeling sorry for them and "saving" them. The payoff for such self-loathing is set out in another prayer of St. Thomas Aquinas: "And I pray that you will lead lead me, a sinner, to the banquet where you, with your Son and Holy Spirit, are true and perfect light, total fulfillment, everlasting joy, gladness without end, and perfect happiness to your saints." With a carrot like this dangling in front of the suffering Christian's nose, it is no wonder that saints were able to endure such self-torture.

Unfortunately, this way of relating to the deity is not confined to the human-to-god bond: all too often, such breast-beating blackmail creeps into human-to-human relationships and contributes to much of the interpersonal stress in marital couples. Each partner, infected with the negative Christian attitude toward self-love, enters the relationship with the self-loathing that is the hallmark of a good Christian, and expects the partner to love him or her for the same self-loathing that is supposed to find such favor with God. People with such low self-esteem often talk glibly about "loving" others while "hating" themselves, in a manner that would, no doubt, please the good Thomas à Kempis. In psychotherapy, the situation is often revealed to be something like this: "I don't like myself, but if I can get so-and-so to love me, then perhaps I can learn to like myself." Each looks for boundless love from the other, and of course each becomes disappointed, since it is impossible to recognize, let alone accept, love from someone else if you do not love yourself. Because of this core of self-loathing, any genuine love the partner does try to show is misinterpreted or else dismissed as inadequate or nongenuine.

One hears a great deal of negative comment these days about something called the "me" generation, which is often equated with a falling away from traditional religious, usually Christian, values. These comments usually come from people who are steeped in the Christian attitudes about self-acceptance and self-esteem. However, we should never forget that the Christian expects to be rewarded for all his or her self-denial in this life with life eternal in the next. With the lure of everlasting life the Christian church has played on the insatiable, infantile, narcissistic greed of the sheep in its flock for centuries. But what could be more greedy, more "me," than to expect more than one's share of existence? And could anything be more immoral than to play on people's infantile greed in this way? As Paul Pruyser has put it, "Pious humility is not submission to the unalterable features of reality, but to the whimsies of a fantasized Father-Creator who is to be charmed while one purports to obey him."[10]

It follows from all this that children growing up in families relatively untainted by Christian notions of self-loathing will be more likely to develop self-esteem than children in a "good" Christian home. However, self-esteem is more than simply an absence of self-hate. For its development it requires an environment in which infants feel loved, and in which children feel that those who love them are accepting of their right to develop according to their own innate timetable, to learn to master the world, including their intrapsychic and interpersonal world, in their own way. But there are many teachings of the Christian church that interfere with these processes, as we will see in subsequent chapters.

NOTES

1. Nathan W. Ackerman. "Preventive Implications of Family Research," in Gerald Caplan, ed., *Prevention of Mental Disorders in Children: Initial Explorations* (New York: Basic Books, 1961), p. 144.

2. Marie Jahoda. *Current Concepts of Positive Mental Health* (New York: Basic Books, 1958), p. 23.

3. Jules Henry, *Pathways to Madness* (London: Jonathan Cape, 1972), p. 374.

4. Solomon Ganzfried, *Code of Jewish Law,* trans. Hyman E. Goldin (New York: Hebrew Publishing Company, 1927), vol 1., chap. 29, p. 92.

5. Thomas à Kempis, *The Imitation of Christ* (Chicago: Moody Press, 1980), p. 27.

6. Ibid., p. 35.

7. Ibid., p. 145.

8. Ibid., p. 157.

9. Ibid., p. 244.

10. Paul Pruyser, *Between Belief and Unbelief* (New York: Harper and Row, 1974), p. 76.

4

Dependency, Interdependency, and Self-Actualization

"Except ye be converted, and become as little children, ye shall not enter into the Kingdom of Heaven."

—Matt. 18:3

"It is not sad to see people growing old: it is only sad to see people growing old without growing up."

—Author Unknown

A child that is welcomed into a family at birth is already well on the road to health. Most of the evidence in support of this statement is empirical and comes from the experience of health care and people service professionals who work with families; however, some well-controlled studies have demonstrated that, in a number of areas, children born to women after they have been refused abortion do not fare as well as the offspring of mothers who had not wanted to terminate the pregnancy.[1]

Whether or not the welcome mat is out for her, the neonate comes into this world with a limited but effective repertoire of techniques for making her needs known, her cry being the main method of communication. One of the first tasks of new parents is to learn this "language," to know when the infant is hungry or sleepy, when she is uncomfortable from a wet diaper, or when the cry is a request for human physical contact. Initally, the infant has no awareness of "mother" or "father"; rather, depending on how her cry is interpreted and how her needs are met, she gradually develops an impression of the world and eventually of the people in it. The interaction patterns that are set up between the infant and parents around the gratification of the infant's needs are crucial for the development of a child's fundamental attitudes to life. Sociologist Jules Henry describes it this way:

> For such empathic absorption of the universe by the baby it is probably better to use "imbue" rather than "teach," for the idea of contact with the universe through another person is not quite captured by the terms "learn" and "teach." When one is imbued in this way—as if sun, water, and time were filtered to one through the body of another person—it becomes difficult to change one's perceptions, for change would be a kind of death—a detachment from the person through whom the universe was absorbed.[2]

Erik Erikson refers to this attitude within the dimensions of basic trust and mistrust. Of this he states: "The general state of trust, furthermore, implies not only that one has learned to rely on the sameness and continuity of the outer providers but also that one may trust oneself and the capacity of one's own organs to cope with urges; that one is able to consider oneself trustworthy enough so that the providers will not need to be on guard or to leave."[3]

In order for the infant to emerge from this stage with a fairly high level of basic trust, the parents must not only learn to interpret her cry correctly and respond to it appropriately, but to do so without undue anxiety about the cry itself. Too much anxiety on the part of parents can lead to attempts to anticipate the infant's needs in order to prevent or minimize the crying; it is important for the infant to cry in order to come to appreciate a connection between her felt need and her crying, and between her cry and the environment's response to her. If her needs are anticipated and met before the infant can express them, her ability to adapt to later stages of development may be severely compromised.

Conversely, if the infant's cry is protracted to the point of exhaustion before she is fed, changed, or cuddled, she will grow up convinced that gratification of needs is always associated with pain. Worse still is the situation in which the parental responses to the infant's cries are random and chaotic, sometimes anticipating, sometimes ignoring, and at other times misinterpreting those cries. With this kind of parenting, the infant will grow up with a profound mistrust of the world, an attitude that will inevitably shape the rest of her development.

How parents deal with infants' biological needs is certainly important; equally important is the manner in which parents deal with their emotional needs. Infants need eye contact as well as vocal and verbal stimulation from caring adults; and they require lots of cuddling, including plenty of skin-to-skin contact. On this latter point, Ashley Montague has stated:

The infant's need for body contact is compelling. If that need is not adequately satisfied, even though all other needs are adequately met, it will suffer. Because the consequences of a lack of satisfaction of such basic needs as hunger, thirst, rest, sleep, bowel and bladder elimination, and avoidance of dangerous and painful stimuli are fairly obvious, we are conscious of the importance of satisfying them. In the case of tactile needs, the consequences of failing to satisfy them are far from obvious, and so these needs have been mostly overlooked.[4]

This is important from the point of view of the development of healthy sexuality, as we shall see in chapter 6.

During this early stage of primary narcissism, the infant is preoccupied with her own needs. From these early experiences with mother and father, however, she learns to differentiate between herself and others who respond to her. The eventual outcome of these interactions is a template on which all subsequent life experiences are built. If her needs are met more or less sensitively, she feels a sense of omnipotence; conversely, if her needs are met in a haphazard fashion, she will feel a sense of impotence or despair.

While the roots of her self-esteem are to be found in these early experiences, the infant's healthy development requires that this narcissistic omnipotence undergo a metamorphosis into a sense of realistic confidence in the world, and a healthy sense of competence in her ability to function in that world. This transition can be either facilitated or discouraged by her parents in two ways: by the manner in which they cope with the frustration of infantile needs and the manner in which they respond to her attempt to self-actualize, to develop a sense of mastery, and adapt to each developmental stage as it comes along.

One view on child rearing, regrettably still held in some circles, is that children grow up because they are forced to by the demands of the real world, and that it is the parents' responsibility to frustrate children's infantile demands when they, the parents, feel it is "time." A competing view holds that children grow up because they want to, that one should not pressure infants to give up the breast or bottle or to become toilet trained but rather let them do it at their own time and in their own way. The first hypothesis assumes that we all grow up reluctantly and incompletely, with an inner deep longing for the security that goes with the state of primary narcissism of the infant at the breast. The very existence of religions is sometimes explained psychologically on the basis of this presumed infantile residue; but the opposite may be more to the point, namely, that religions actively foster the perpetuation of primary narcissism in human beings.

As with most extreme positions, the truth probably lies somewhere in between. It is certainly true that the love demonstrated by parents in their multitudinous acts of nurturance and affectionate play, coupled with the sensitivity and appropriateness with which they frustrate children's infantile wishes and demands, do play a major role in determining how children feel about themselves throughout their lives. But the developing child is far from passive clay in the hands of the parents.

Most modern students of child development hold that children grow up largely because they are driven from inside to master their inner and outer worlds. This view postulates that within the individual child is an ever present pressure to self-actualize, to realize her adaptive potential to the fullest. From a very early age, the child struggles to master the inanimate and the interpersonal environment and manifests a great deal of obvious pleasure when she succeeds. That mastery is different from control. Control is more akin to the old infantile omnipotence of the narcissistic stage, whereas mastery implies a capacity to cope with both successes and disappointments in an adaptive way. The more successes the child has in mastering the environment, the more she experiences a sense of competence,[5] a subjective state that enhances her self-esteem. By the time the child grows to adolescence, the interpersonal environment becomes as important as the physical environment. How to say hello to a boy or work with her teammates on the basketball team assumes the importance once occupied by her preoccupation with learning to ride a bicycle. Thus, interpersonal competence becomes a major source of adult self-esteem.

Parents cannot initiate any of these active steps the child takes in the service of her own growth, but they can, due to ignorance, insensitivity, or both, retard the process in a variety of ways. Consider this scenario. An older infant, being spoon-fed by her mother, reaches out to grab the spoon in an attempt to learn to feed herself. One mother may recognize this as an important milestone and be prepared to tolerate the mess, delay, and inconvenience that follow if she goes along with the child's wishes. Another mother might resist and insist on continuing to feed the child herself in the interests of efficiency and cleanliness. In such instances the struggle for mastery may be thwarted, and the child's emotional reactions misinterpreted by the mother as evidence that she is an ungrateful little girl. The seeds of conflict are sown.

In a second scenario, a six-year-old boy is eagerly trying to put together a new toy truck his father has given him, but is expressing some frustration in the process. The boy's mother, interpreting his struggles as a plea for her to intervene, takes over the task without asking her son if he wants her help or not. This intervention evokes a violent temper tantrum from the child, who promptly gives up in his attempt to master the challenge posed by the truck. Mother is confused. We can only speculate about her motives. Her tendency to be overprotective made it difficult for her to tolerate any frustration in the child; she tended to react to her son's distress in this situation in the same manner as she responded to his cry for food as an infant.

Parental interference with a child's self-actualization may stem from the opposite concern, namely, a fear that initiative is not being shown in those areas where and when parents feel it should be. Each individual matures physically according to his or her own inner timetable. In the area of self-actualization, each individual unfolds in a similarly stepwise fashion, and parents can make this unfolding difficult by imposing their notions of what that timetable should be. A young girl of fifteen may not be ready for dating boys in spite of the fact that her mother, who dated at fourteen, thinks her daughter ought to be well into this stage. In a variety of ways she may communicate her anxiety to her daughter, who begins to feel there is something wrong with her; her self-esteem begins to suffer, making it difficult for her to start this phase of her life at sixteen according to the dictates of her own inner timetable.

The task of being parents is, in many ways, like a balancing act in the circus. On the one hand, parents should do their sensitive best to meet the growing child's needs for nurturance. On the other hand, they should not discourage the processes of individuation and self-actualization, by which the child becomes aware of her essential autonomy from her parents, with her own unique feelings, ambitions, and identity. Where families are successful in this balancing act, individuals emerge into adult life with what Helm Stierlin has called a high degree of "related individuation." This term refers to an ability to relate openly and to communicate congruently with others while at the same time experiencing a strong sense of self and a high level of self esteem. Where parents fail in the balancing act, we find over-individuation and under-individuation. Stierlin et al. describe these two states:

> Over-individuation sets too rigid and impenetrable boundaries: independence turns into isolation and separateness into bleak solitude; communication with others fails.
>
> Under-individuation, however, means the boundaries are ineffective—too soft, porous, penetrable and brittle. Diminished individuation may lead to fusion and absorption into other, stronger organisms.[6]

Many people in our society appear to share in the myth that individuation and self-actualization involve a state where one stoically abjures the need for close contact with and support of others. In actual fact, the truth is quite the opposite. As Stierlin et al. point out, "Progress in individuation demands, therefore, ever new levels of communication and reconciliation." For them, the term "related individuation" expresses "a general principle that a higher level of individuation both requires and allows a higher level of relatedness."[7]

CHRISTIAN DOCTRINE AND RELATED INDIVIDUATION

Jesus is reported to have preached, "Whosoever therefore shall humble himself as this little child, the same is greatest in the Kingdom of Heaven" (Matt. 18:4). Whatever Jesus himself meant by that statement, his followers took it literally, and when it came time to found a terrestrial institution, they developed a set of teachings that promoted infantile dependency in their followers as it discouraged adult interdependency and mature self-reliance. In order to appreciate how Christian doctrine discourages adult-related individuation, we need to examine Christianity's response to three aspects of human behavior: anxiety, ambivalence, and human communication.

Christianity and Anxiety

Anxiety can be defined as a painful feeling of apprehension, fear, or dread at any time when one's integrity is threatened, and the individual feels incompetent to deal with the threat. The threat may emanate from internal sources such as the anticipated punishment or loss of approval from a loved one in response to thoughts, feelings, or behavior deemed unacceptable; the threat may come from outside as fear of realistic dangers or the existential dread associated with ultimate mortality. It varies in intensity from individual to individual and from time to time within the same person. When very intense, as in so-called panic attacks, anxiety is accompanied by physiological symptoms such as rapid heart beat, increased respiration, and other signs of heightened sympathetic nervous activity.

Erik Erikson makes an important point about anxiety: "Much of what we ascribe to neurotic *anxiety* and much of what we ascribe to existential *dread* is really only man's distinctive form of *fear:* for, as an animal, for the sake of survival, scans near and far with specialized senses fit for a special environment, man must scan both his inner and his outer environment for indications of permissible activity and for promises of identity."[8]

While neurotic anxiety and existential dread may be similar, there are nevertheless many differences which need to be recognized. Existential dread, the fear of the unknown, often aroused at the comprehension of the essential mysteries of the universe, is a feeling that could be used as a stimulus to promote bonds between human beings. This is not the case in our Christian society, which tends to anthropomorphize the unknown and to encourage the anxious human being to grovel on his or her knees before it.

Much so-called neurotic anxiety is generated in human relationships and the more troublesome the human relationships are, the more difficult it is for bonds to be formed between people, connections that would enable them to live in an adaptive human way with the essential mystery of life. Freud put it this way:

> We are threatened with suffering from three directions: from our own body, which is doomed to decay and dissolution and which cannot even do without pain and anxiety as warning signals; from the external world, which may rage against us with overwhelming and merciless forces of destruction; and finally from our relations to other men. The suffering which comes from this last source is perhaps more painful to us than any other.[9]

To recapitulate, individuals become anxious when they feel unable to cope with a particular situation confronting them. How someone responds to such situations depends on a number of factors, the chief ones being the nature of the threat and the intensity of the reaction to it. More important still is the individual's habitual pattern of dealing with adaptational challenges. If a person has been encouraged in the past to retreat from such challenges and not to seek human support in meeting them, he or she is likely to regress to self-punitive withdrawal or into actual physical symptoms and illness behavior.

Since anxiety is a signal that the adaptational ability of the individual is being or is about to be challenged, it can function as a stimulus to mastery resulting in enhanced self-esteem, or else as a blow resulting in failure and loss of self-esteem. The latter is more likely to happen if the anxiety is intense and if human supports are lacking or ineffective. Under these circumstances, the individual retreats into himself and away from human contact, falling back on more infantile coping strategies to deal with the anxiety-provoking situation. The more regressed and isolated he becomes, the more damaged his self-esteem, and thus the more likely he is to fall for the pitch of the religious huckster of whatever stripe. When that happens, the individual becomes locked into a situation that may make him feel better momentarily, but in the long run may make it impossible for him to develop further adult problem-solving abilities.

According to Christian doctrine and liturgy, adaptational challenges associated with anxiety are not to be resolved by using one's human support system to help develop a higher level of coping skills. Such feelings should be suppressed or denied. One Christian psychologist, John A. Hammes, put it bluntly: "Not only should needless anxiety be avoided. Other unhealthy emotional responses should be resisted. This means avoiding hate, anger, jealousy, envy, bitterness, and depression. . . . For the Christian, however, indulgence in such moods indicates a lack of trust in divine providence."[10]

If such denial is impossible, the anxious Christian is encouraged to regress to a dependent symbiotic state with the great anthropomorphized unknown and unknowable. A prayer in the Anglican prayer book titled "For Those in Anxiety" teaches this message specifically: "Almighty God, who art afflicted in the afflictions of thy people; regard with tender compassion those in anxiety and distress; bear their sorrows and cares; supply all their manifold needs; and help them and us to put our whole trust and confidence in thee; through Jesus Christ our Lord. Amen." Note that the prayer does not ask God to help the anxious and distressed to maximize their human support systems in order that they might bear their own burdens and learn and grow thereby. It says nothing about asking God to enlighten the anxious and distressed as to the sources of their suffering, and to enhance their problem-solving skills by tackling those problems that can be solved. It says nothing about asking God to help the anxious and distressed develop confidence in themselves; rather, it urges the supplicant not to make the effort, but rather to "put our whole trust and confidence" in God.

In Phil. 2:13 we find doctrinal support for this liturgical approach: "For it is God which worketh in you both to will and to do of his good pleasure." In the Lord's Prayer, the supplicant says, "Thy will be done." With this line of doctrine, the Christian church explicitly promotes under-individuation by preaching that it is wrong for human beings to use their own innate drive toward mastery and self-actualization. In times of stress, the Christian is expected to fuse with and become absorbed with the stronger organism, God. In promoting this attitude, the church is like the overanxious mother, who, taking over completely, robbed her son of the opportunity to learn when he was frustrated by the toy truck.

One of the most difficult adaptational tasks we human beings face is confronting our own mortality and facing the fact that life is short, often painful, frequently frightening, and for many people patently unfair. It is difficult for human beings to come to terms with these existential facts without being consumed with rage or overwhelmed with despair. However, it is not difficult to understand how the Christian church has been so successful in its manipulation of human infantile greed with the promise of life after death —by teaching that suffering is simply God's way of testing the faithful for their fitness to be with him throughout eternity. Nothing demonstrates the consummate political skill of the church fathers more than the myths they developed to "help" adherents cope with these existential problems. It is little wonder that, in the absence of more mutually supportive, humanistically oriented options, so many people continue to embrace those myths.

The notion that one can have more than one's share of existence is an irresistible sales pitch. In the early centuries of the church's existence, Christians mobilized the despair and discontent of the poor and the socially disenfranchised people throughout the Roman Empire with promises of much more than the bread and circuses offered by the wealthy; they promised life everlasting. Having convinced the masses that this prize would be theirs if they embraced Christianity, the early fathers assured success to the new religion.

In our own day, it is not only the poor, the unsophisticated, and the uneducated in whom infantile greed is aroused and stimulated by the doctrine of life after death. A medical colleague and friend of mine, a seemingly happy family man, once told me, while I was visiting his home, that he would commit suicide instantly if he were to be convinced that there was no life after death. I shuddered to think of the impact this statement must have had on his children grouped around him; one can only conjecture what it communicated to the children about their own meaning and value to their father. In a lecture on bioethics I heard some years ago, the speaker declared that death had no or little meaning unless we believed that we were God's creatures who would one day find perfect happiness.[10]

Infantile narcissistic greed is alive and well and apparently thrives in medical academia. Few people have recognized that while the church was declaring gluttony to be one of the seven deadly sins, it was fostering greed in its followers with promises of streets of gold and Elysian fields.

Christianity purports to relieve existential dread with its claim of a kind, loving father who banished death for human beings by sacrificing his only son on a cross, and who guarantees us a life everlasting if we only buy the product the church is selling. Unfortunately, many of the elements of that product tend to reinforce the difficulties human beings have in relating to each other. If Jesus Christ is the true source of our strength, how can we possibly develop human-to-human relationships that would be supportive rather than the source of suffering which is, in Freud's words, "perhaps more painful to us than any other"?

Christianity and Ambivalence

Much of the pain in interpersonal relationships stems from the existence of ambivalence or, more properly, the manner in which human beings are socialized to deal with what has been defined in one recently published psychiatric textbook as "the presence of strong and often overwhelming simultaneous contrasting attitudes, ideas, feelings, and drives toward an object, person or goal."[11] While a child's capacity to deal with such mixed feelings is quite limited, one of the main characteristics of a healthy adult is the ability to accept that ambivalence is a part of all human relationships and to tolerate the discomfort associated with ambivalence without resorting to maladaptive, inappropriate behavior.

During his early omnipotent narcissistic stage of development, the infant is considered to be in a pre-ambivalent stage, with little awareness of a distinction between himself and the outside world, and no recognition of painful feelings if his needs are met in a reasonably sensitive fashion. As individuation develops, infantile omnipotent narcissism begins to make way, hopefully, for a sense of competence in dealing with the outside world. The child not only becomes aware of those around him as individuals distinct from himself; he also comes to appreciate that, depending on the nature of the interaction with them, he has both pleasant and unpleasant feelings connected with his contacts with others at various times. The child is also distressed to discover in himself that he feels a sense of impotent rage toward the mother for whom he feels such warmth and love whenever she frustrates him. Erik Erikson has postulated that this move from the pre-ambivalent narcissistic stage to the real world of human interaction, however gradual, has cosmic overtones. Erikson terms this a "psychic fall from grace,"[12] which prompts the intriguing hypothesis concerning the origins of the Hebrew creation myth. The Garden of Eden may very well represent a cosmic projection of the stage of pre-ambivalent narcissism; the ejection from the Garden would then represent the move out of this blissful state into a world in which all must struggle, however unsuccessfully, with ambivalence.

The more the infant recognizes that the frustrating mother and the gratifying mother are one and the same person, the more acute becomes the adaptational challenge of dealing with these ambivalent feelings. Another potential source of frustration stems from the child's emerging need to develop mastery. Although he struggles to achieve a sense of competence through his own efforts, this struggle runs counter to the child's still remembered state of narcissistic bliss. As one group of psychoanalysts have put it, "No person, however, at least unconsciously, completely gives up his longing to enjoy magical dependence on the delegated omnipotence of the mother."[13] If the infant's crude attempts at mastery are not supported—or, worse still, frustrated—by the caring adults around him, the more rage is generated, the more regression is encouraged, and the more difficult the resolution of ambivalence becomes.

A major factor in determining a child's success in resolving ambivalence concerns how caring adults react to his struggles with negative emergency affects. If the parents become punitive in the face of the child's expressions of rage, using emotional withdrawal, guilt-inducing responses, or even physical punishment, they may seriously compromise his emotional growth. If they put appropriate limits on the child's behavior when he is under the influence of his negative feelings (as in a temper tantrum), but refrain from communicating that he is bad to have such feelings, they are increasing the chance that he will develop reasonably healthy techniques for dealing with anger and ambivalence.

Successful resolution of ambivalent feelings toward loved ones is an essential factor in the development of adult self-esteem; failure to do so is characteristic of all forms of psychiatric illness. Usually this failure takes the form of patients' consciously professing—to themselves and others—unalloyed "love" toward, say, a parent, even while engaging in distancing, passive-aggressive, or self-punitive behavior. I have never ceased to be amazed at the number of young adult patients who claim to love their parents completely, yet who never visit them, even though they live only a few blocks away. Suicidal patients, who profess nothing hut love for their parents, are always shocked when told that if they were not also enraged at their parents, they would hardly have tried to kill one of their parents' children. In other instances, the ambivalent feelings turn wholly negative: the parent is all bad with no redeeming features whatever.

In examining how Christian doctrine shapes people's attitudes regarding ambivalence, it is worth remembering that Christianity has many roots in Judaic law, integral to which was the codification of human feelings. According to that code, "Anger is likewise an extremely bad vice, and it is proper that one should keep away from it, and he should accustom himself not to get angry even at things that he needs to become angry."[14] Elsewhere, a man is reminded that he should "neither be gay and jocular nor should he be morose and melancholy, but he should be happy."[15] The Jewish code has strict rules about attitudes toward parents which are appropriated by Christianity: "Even if his father be wicked and a sinner, it is proper for him [i.e., the son], nevertheless, to honor and to fear him."[16]

An examination of Christian doctrine and teachings leaves one convinced that it would be very difficult for a true Christian to grow up enough to come to terms with normal human ambivalence. In a number of scriptural passages Christians are warned explicitly not to attempt to do so: "A double-minded man is unstable in all ways" (James 1:8). "Out of the same mouth proceedeth blessing and cursing. My brethren, these things ought not to be" (James 3:10). "Draw nigh to God, and he will draw nigh to you. Cleanse your hands, ye sinners: and purify your hearts, ye double minded" (James 4:8).

Simplistic childish dichotomies permeate the entire structure of doctrinal Christianity. Indeed, it might be said that this structure is based on such dichotomies: God and the devil, heaven and hell, sin and salvation. By its very nature Christianity requires adherents to think in terms of black and white, never shades of grey, and most certainly never in color. The true Christian must always be in a state of torment, since he can never be really certain that God has forgiven him for his deeply felt negative feelings, despite the Catholic confessional and the fundamentalist trick of self-deception known as being "saved" or "born again." Paul said, "For all have sinned and come short of the glory of God" (Rom. 3:2). In James we read, "For whosoever shall keep the whole law, and yet offend in one point, he is guilty of all" (James 2:10). How's that for justice?

Christian Doctrine and Communication

The mechanism of well-functioning human-to-human relationships depend on sound negotiation skills, oiled by congruent communication. This occurs when an individual speaks her thoughts freely, expresses her feelings openly but discriminatingly and appropriately, and behaves in accordance with stated attitudes and beliefs and expressed feelings. Roughly speaking, we communicate in two ways: verbally and nonverbally. Nonverbal communication takes place along a number of channels: neurophysiological reactions (sighing, crying, etc.); gestures and behavior ("body language"); and nonverbal vocalization (tone, dialect, etc.). Nonverbal communication is analogic in nature and more primitive developmentally. Verbal communication is digital* and symbolic in nature, uses more advanced neurological structures and pathways, and appears later in the development of the individual.

All communication involving a dyad or group is circular. A message from *A* is received by *B,* who responds to that message in some way. Even a stony silence is a response; one cannot *not* communicate in a dyad or group. *B*'s response becomes then a message for *A,* whose response in turn becomes a second message to *B,* and so on. Communication is congruent when the nonverbal are in harmony with the verbal messages.

There is a link between how individuals communicate and how they function internally. Adult human beings function in six interrelated modes: *perceptual* (seeing, hearing, and feeling); *cognitive* (thinking, reasoning, and conceptualizing); *affective* (feeling); *biological* (e.g., breathing, perspiring, and digesting); *behavioral* (doing and acting); and *verbal* (speaking). When all the modes are in harmony with one another, we may assume that functioning is optimal, and that the communication with others will be congruent. Under these circumstances not only do people speak their minds, express their feelings relatively openly, and behave according to their stated attitudes and beliefs, but their autonomic nervous systems function in a smooth and integrated fashion. When confronted with such congruent communicators, we tend to think of them as "open," "genuine," and as "having their act together."[17]

The newborn has highly vocal but only primitive and nonverbal means of responding to inner events. As the child matures, she develops an awareness of a connection between her cries and the parental response to them, and thereby learns that she can influence the environment in this way. At the same time, she is struggling to make sense out of the messages she receives from her parents: the tone of her mother's voice, her frowns, or the way the child's father looks at her when he holds her. As neurological develop-

---

*This term is used in neuropsychological literature to denote the difference between verbal and nonverbal communication.

ment proceeds, she develops the ability to imitate parental words, and language enters the developmental picture. As the child's verbal facility increases, she learns to put into words what is happening to her in the various modes of her functioning: "I want to go to the bathroom" and "I am mad at you, Mommy."

If her parents are congruent communicators, the child's chances of developing in a way that promotes modal harmony within herself and congruent communication with others is enhanced. As Theodore Lidz puts it, "Here he [the child] learns how effective words will be; whether they concur with unspoken communications; whether they are apt to match the feelings that accompany them; whether they subserve problem solving or are just as often a means of masking the existence of problems."[18]

However, fully congruent communication is difficult for most people in the Western world. Pointing out that nonverbal communication refers to inner events, whereas verbal communications refers to external events, Jurgen Reusch argues that for the average Westerner, "the vocabulary for events occurring inside the organism and referring to bodily experience is rudimentary."[19] René Spitz makes the same point:

> Average Western man has elected to emphasize in his culture diacritic perception both in regard to communication with others and with himself. Introspection is discounted as unwholesome and frowned upon, so that we are hardly conscious of what goes on in us unless we are sick. Our deeper sensations do not reach our awareness, do not become meaningful to us; we ignore and repress their messages. Indeed we are fearful of them and we betray this fear in many ways.[20]

Whether or not there are any developmental or biological reasons for this discrepancy, Christianity has had a powerful tendency to make people phobic about congruent verbal communication of feelings. This observation has been made by Christians themselves. One cleric, in trying to understand why Christians "break down," wrote, "There seems to have been in the church a tendency to stifle the expression of real personal feelings (for instance anger, ecstasy, despair, grief) and to encourage a consistent 'neutral pleasantness' as the proper way to express oneself."[21]

Because Christianity frowns on pleasure and promotes suffering as a desirable end, it is difficult for Christians and those influenced by Christian teachings to express the welfare affects of joy and happiness. Emergency affects such as anger (one of the seven deadly sins) are explicitly discouraged in Christian teachings, "For the wrath of man worketh not the righteousness of God" (James 1:20). For some Christians, the verbal expression of anger is an offense which calls for physical violence against the culprit. An Ontario Baptist minister was charged with child abuse for leaving bruises on his eight-

month-old child, whom he spanked with a wooden spoon for being "angry."
The minister pleaded with his fellow fundamentalists to come to his aid on
the grounds that the authority of the Bible ("spare the rod and spoil the
child") was being challenged in a secular court.[22]

Anger, although often an unpleasant feeling, is a normal human emotion,
a response to frustration of one kind or another. In the Christian tradition,
the tendency is to train children from an early age to believe that only bad,
evil people feel angry. Such an attitude generates intense conflict between
what the child *actually* feels and what he *should* feel in order to be accepted
by the adult caretakers. Such conflicts are intensified if the child witnesses
violent physical outbursts by adults, especially if that violence is directed at
the child himself. To spank a child with a wooden spoon because he expressed
anger verbally transmits a very dangerous and confusing message, namely,
that it is all right to use physical violence but not to express anger verbally.
No wonder the Christian record is so bloody.

Conflicts of this sort generate anxiety, another painful emotion. To avoid
this feeling, we humans develop what are called defense mechanisms, attitudinal
and behavioral responses designed to ward off the unacceptable feelings that
give rise to anxiety. To prevent the painful anxiety from emerging, the child
may deny that he is angry at his mother but vent his anger on a younger
sibling or the family dog (displacement). He may bend over backwards to
demonstrate that he is not angry at his mother and become oversolicitous
and attentive (reaction-formation). Or else, the child may deal with his anger
at his father by convincing himself that it is his father who is angry at him
(projection).

Defenses may work for a time to protect the individual from anxiety,
but they eventually "break down," with the result that the unacceptable feelings
erupt into awareness. This eruption may be associated with the production
of "symptoms" that may lead to the need for medical or psychiatric intervention;
or it may result in disharmony in relationships since the individual concerned
has never been trained to deal with such emergency emotions in a manner
not destructive to the human-to-human bond. At times the breakthrough of
angry feelings may take the form of a violent, antisocial act, thereby reinforcing
the Christian notion that anger itself is evil. In reality, it is the lessons people
learn about anger in our "Christian" society that are at the bottom of problems with anger.

One modern Christian counselor reveals the church's continuing attitude
toward anger when she advises that this affect can best be handled in psychotherapy with religious patients "through the use of introspection, reflection, insight, rearrangement of presuppositions, and giving feedback to the
offender" (my italics).[23] As a way of dealing with anger, Christian psychologist John Hammes advises his readers to release the tension through physical

recreation: "Is is difficult to be angry after swimming fifty yards, running as mile, or doing thirty push-ups." Hammes says nothing, however, about trying to confront the person with whom one is angry for the purpose of resolving the issue; in fact, Hammes suggests that his "solution" to feeling angry would lead one to be "thankful" that the "aggression" had not been directed against a human "target."[24] Hammes thus reveals himself as a product of a belief system that has succeeded in making human beings terrified of their normal natural emergency affects.

The Christian influence in discouraging human-to-human supports is neither indirect nor subtle. Thomas à Kempis's *The Imitation of Christ* contains upwards of twenty explicit warnings about the futility of trusting other human beings to be a source of support. At times, one seems to tempt the wrath of God by daring to lean on one's fellow creatures: "Thou oughtest to be so dead to such affections of beloved friends, that, as much as concerns thee, thou shouldest wish to be without all company of men. Man approacheth so much the nearer unto God, the further off he departeth from all earthly consolation."[25] With this kind of indoctrination operating in good Christians for centuries, it is not too difficult to understand why people in our society have so much trouble getting along with each other.

Prayer

While promoting a distrust of human-to-human communication and support, the Christian church encourages human-to-god communication, commonly called prayer.

William James, who called prayer "the very soul and essence of religion,"[26] insisted that the phenomenon of prayer was not open to scientific scrutiny: "If we take the word [prayer] in the wider sense as meaning every kind of inward communion or conversation with the power recognized as divine, we can easily see that scientific criticism leaves it untouched."[27] James's statement turns out to be prophetic, since the psychology of religion has to this day failed to deal with the subject of prayer; as Paul Pruyser has indicated, the psychologist's "curiosity" was tempered by his "reverence."[28] However, this "very soul and essence of religion" demonstrates how Christianity tends to reduce its adherents to the state of abjectly whining, cajolingly coercive infants, whether the goal of the particular entreaty is good weather, relief of pain, the welfare of the souls of the dear departed, or laying up grace in heaven.

The phenomenon of prayer enables us to make a link between the Christian concept of God and that of Eastern mystical religion. At first glance, there seems to be little in common between the set prayers repeated week after week by mainline Christian denominations and the act of meditation by the mystic, who seeks in a quiet, contemplative manner to relate to the universal Other. The mystical religious approach to God relies heavily on a losing of self in an attempt to effect a union with the infinite. This is not something that is encouraged in organized Christianity. As the GAP (Group for the Advancement of Psychiatry) report on mysticism states: "The purposes of organized religions are multifarious, but providing unmediated awareness of the 'divine milieu' is a minor one, if not one to be dismissed altogether."[29] The Christian relates to God in a manner determined by those who are "trained" to know what the Bible "means" and what God really "wants." In both approaches to this communion with the divinity, the communication is of the one-way variety; a real problem is posed to the Christian church if one of its adherents claims that the communication has been two-way. The question in these instances is whether to build a shrine on the spot or have the poor soul transported to the nearest mental hospital.

The most destructive aspect of both prayer and meditation is that they discourage the development of human-to-human communication skills as well as the formation of human support groups to aid in solving those problems that can be solved and coping adaptively with those existential problems that cannot. If the true Christian obeys Paul's instructions to carry on a monologue with God "without ceasing," it will be pretty difficult to learn how to make human relationships work. The traditional religious solution to the painfulness of human-to-human interaction—prayer and meditation—continues to perpetuate relationship patterns that encourage people to break off their attempts to develop a high level of relationship skills and make them regress to religious "solutions." It is much easier, after all, to talk to a God who doesn't talk back than it is to carry on a dialogue with those human beings closest to us. If the energy now used in trying to promote one-way communication to God were rechanneled into educational programs to promote skills in two-way human communication, negotiation, and mutual support, we might all be pleasantly amazed at the improvement in human relationships.

The disruption of human interpersonal relationships, one of the key features of all forms of psychiatric illness, is the topic of a current chicken-and-egg debate. Does the biologically determined illness cause the rift, or is the rift the result of poor relationship skills in a society where people are given more encouragement to bare their bosoms to the almighty than to be open with those humans closest to them?

A couple of clinical examples will illustrate the conflict between human-to-human and human-to-God communication.

A young schizophrenic woman stated in a family therapy session that whenever she found herself getting upset at home, not being able to talk with her father, she would go to her mother. The mother would then go to the father, who always reacted by gathering the family to kneel in the living room while he prayed aloud to God. The patient stated that she liked these sessions because when her father was praying to God, he said things about her that he was apparently unable to say to her directly. In this way she found out that he cared for her.

In another family, the young son was the identified patient; in one session I conducted, he began crying at a certain point in the interview and kept looking at his parents for some kind of human response. The father, a classic example of the stereotypical emotionally inarticulate male, stared off into space looking very tense. The mother closed her eyes and sat quietly in the chair. When I asked her what was going on inside her, she replied that she was praying to God to help the family. The mother's one-way conversation with God, however, was clearly not what her son needed at that point in time.

CHRISTIANITY'S PROMOTION OF INFANTILE BEHAVIOR

Many psychoanalytical studies have pointed to the tendency of religions in general, and Christianity in particular, to encourage infantile dependency while discouraging related individuation, to use Stierlin's phrase. Edith Weisskopf-Joelson states: "In a society where independence is a high value, dependency needs can be satisfied, for example, by neurotic avenues such as illness, by semi-neurotic avenues such as acquiring an excessive number of college degrees to postpone maturity, or by highly acceptable avenues such as satisfying children's dependency needs and, then, getting vicarious enjoyment from their satisfaction. But the royal road to dependency are religious faiths."[30] Commenting on Freud's views, Paul Pruyser puts it this way, "Religion is a stylized and socially acceptable way of resisting nature's demand for growing up."[31] Erik Erikson has made somewhat the same point: "All religions have in common the periodical childlike surrender to a Provider or providers who dispense earthly fortune as well as spiritual health; the demonstration of one's smallness and dependence through the medium of reduced posture and humble gesture."[32]

Indeed, Christianity is among of the most powerful contributors to a feeling of helplessness and worthlessness in children exposed to its doctrine. Martin Seligman has summed up the evidence from the scientific literature on the role of learned helplessness in the development of children:

> I am convinced that certain arrangements of environmental contingencies will produce a child who believes he is helpless—that he cannot succeed—and that other contingencies will produce a child who believes that his responses matter—that he can control his little world. If a child believes he is helpless he will perform stupidly, regardless of his IQ. If a child believes he is helpless, he will not write piano sonatas, regardless of his inherent musical genius. On the other hand, if

a child believes that he has control and mastery, he may outperform more talented peers who lack such a belief.[33]

No more serious charge can be made against the Christian church than that it actively discourages its adherents in their attempts to develop into self-reliant adult human beings; and nowhere is there better evidence to back up this charge than in the following Anglican prayer, which is recited each Sunday: "Almighty and most merciful Father, we have erred and strayed from thy way like lost sheep. We have followed the devices and desires of our own hearts. We have offended against Thy holy laws. We have left undone those things which we ought to have done and we have done those things which we ought not to have done; and there is no health in us. But thou, oh Lord, have mercy on us, miserable offenders, etc." It is hard to imagine a process less designed to develop healthy adult capacity for related individuation than for someone to pray Sunday after Sunday for God to forgive him for following "the devices and desires of our own hearts." If there were a God, would he not be responsible for planting those "devices and desires"; and if they weren't to be followed, why would he have put them there? One of the hymns of the Anglican/United Church Hymn Book goes: "When I survey the wondrous cross, on which the Prince of glory died, my richest gain I count but lost, and pour contempt on all my pride. Forbid it, Lord, that I should boast, save in the death of Christ, my God: all the vain things that charm me most, I sacrifice them to his blood" (Hymn 109). In another hymn appears the phrase, "I yield my powers to thy command" (Hymn 141).

Erich Fromm has put the problem in a nutshell when he states: "To understand realistically and soberly how limited our power is, is an essential part of wisdom and of maturity; to worship it is masochistic and self-destructive. The one is humility, the other self humiliation."[34]

The power of Christian doctrine to exert control over the lives of those affected by it does not reside solely in its tendency to discourage related individuation and to encourage infantile dependency. Its attitude toward healthy pleasure and its use of the exploitative potential of human guilt has given Christianity further leverage to achieve its goals.

NOTES

1. Wendell W. Watters, *Compulsory Parenthood: The Truth about Abortion* (Toronto: McClelland and Stewart, 1976).

2. Jules Henry, *Pathways to Madness* (London: Jonathan Cape, 1972), p. 60.

3. Erik H. Erickson, "Identity and the Life Cycle," *Psychological Issues* 1, no 1 = Monograph No. 1 (New York: International Universities Press Inc., 1959), p. 61.

4. Ashley Montague, *Touching: The Human Significance of the Skin,* 2d ed. (New York: Harper and Row, 1978), p. 192.

5. Robert W. White, "Ego and Reality in Psychoanalytic Theory," *Psychological Issues* 3, no 3 = Monograph No. 11 (New York: International Universities Press Inc., 1963).

6. Helm Stierlin, Ingeborg Rucker-Emden, Norbert Wetzel, and Michael Wirsching, *The First Interview with the Family* (New York: Brunner-Mazel, 1980), p. 16.

7. Ibid.

8. Erik H. Erickson, *Insight and Responsibility* (New York: W. W. Norton and Company Inc., 1964), p. 103.

9. Sigmund Freud, *Civilization and Its Discontents,* in James Strachey, trans. and ed., *The Complete Psychological Works of Sigmund Freud* (London: Hogarth Press, 1961), 21: 77.

10. John A. Hammes, *Humanistic Psychology: A Christian Interpretation* (New York: Grune and Stratton, 1971), p. 127.

11. Alfred M. Freedman, Harold I. Kaplan, and Benjamin J. Sadock, eds., *Comprehensive Textbook of Psychiatry,* 2d ed. (Baltimore, Md.: The Williams and Wilkins Company, 1975), 2: 2574.

12. Erickson, *Insight and Responsibility,* p. 120.

13. Abram Kardiner, Aaron Karush, and Lionel Ovesey, "A Methodological Study of Freudian Theory," *International Journal of Psychiatry* 2, no 5 (September 1966): 513.

14. Solomon Ganzfried, *Code of Jewish Law,* trans. Hyman E. Goldin (New York: Hebrew Publishing Company, 1927), vol 1, chap. 29, p. 92.

15. Ibid, p. 93.

16. Ibid., vol. 4, chap. 43, p. 2.

17. W. W. Watters, A. Bellissimo, and J. S. Rubenstein, "Teaching Individual Psychotherapy: Learning Objectives in Communication," *Canadian Journal of Psychiatry* 27, no 4 (June 1982): 263–69.

18. Theodore Lidz, *The Person* (New York: Basic Books, Inc, 1968), pp, 205–206.

19. Jurgen Ruesch, "Communication and Psychiatry," in *Comprehensive Textbook of Psychiatry,* 1: 341.

20. René A. Spitz, *The First Year of Life* (New York: International Universities Press, 1965), p. 136.

21. William A. Miller, *Why Do Christians Break Down* (Minneapolis, Minn.: Augsburg Publishing House, 1973), p. 136.

22. "Preacher Fights Back over Charge of Spanking," *The Globe and Mail* (Toronto), October 23, 1987, p. A3.

23. Carole A. Rayburn, "The Religious Patient's Initial Encounter with Psychotherapy," in E. Mark Stern, ed., *Psychotherapy and the Religiously Committed Patient* (New York: The Haworth Press, 1985), p. 42.

24. Hammes, *Humanistic Psychology: A Christian Interpretation,* p. 127.

25. Thomas à Kempis, *The Imitation of Christ* (Chicago: Moody Press, 1980), pp. 219–20.

26. William James, *The Varieties of Religious Experience* (New York: New American Library, 1958), p. 352.

27. Ibid, p. 352.

28. Paul W. Pruyser, "Some Trends in the Psychology of Religion," in H. Newton Malony, ed., *Current Perspectives in the Psychology of Religion* (Grand Rapids, Mich.: William B. Eerdmans Publishing Company, 1977), p. 68.

29. *Mysticism: Spiritual Quest or Psychic Disorders,* Report of the Group of the Advancement of Psychiatry, Committee on Psychiatry and Religion, vol. 9, no. 97 (November 1976).

30. Edith Weisskopf-Joelson, "The Therapeutic Ingredients in Religion and Political Philosophies," in Paul W. Sharkey, ed., *Philosophy, Religion and Psychotherapy* (Washington, D.C.: University Press of America, 1982), p. 193.

31. Paul W. Pruyser, *Between Belief and Unbelief* (New York: Harper and Row, 1974), p. 77.

32. Erik H. Erickson, "Identity and the Life Cycle," p. 65.

33. Martin E. P. Seligman, *Helplessness: On Depression, Development and Death* (San Francisco: W. H. Freeman and Company, 1975), p. 136.

34. Erich Fromm, *Psychoanalysis and Religion* (New Haven, Conn.: Yale University Press, 1950), p. 53.

5

Pleasure, Suffering, and Guilt

"The compulsion to kill pleasure, however, is an undiagnosed illness, endemic in Western culture, emerging now in one form, now in another."
—Jules Henry[1]

"Suffer with Christ, and for Christ, if thou desirest to reign with Christ."
—Thomas à Kempis[2]

The word "pleasure" in Western society carries with it a connotation that is suspect, as if too much pleasure were harmful in some ill-defined way. The fact that pleasure and its role in human behavior are largely ignored in behavioral science literature may be taken as a measure of our collective social phobia about the topic.

Pleasure should be differentiated from entertainment. In fact, it could be argued that a deeply rooted conflict about genuine human pleasure and a limited capacity for experiencing it, may contribute to the overwhelming success of the entertainment "industry." People spend vast amounts of money for the dubious privilege of being allowed to experience life vicariously, making actors, actresses, and rock stars wealthy in the process.

For Freud, the gratification of instinctual impulses constituted not only the main source of pleasure, but also the raw material out of which the personality developed. The "pleasure principle" was the only governor of the infant's behavior; this behavior was gradually modified in response to the so-called reality principle, which was always in direct opposition to the pleasure principle.[3] The demands of reality led to more and more frustration of instinctual needs, accompanied by a variety of emergency emotions such as rage and

75

disappointment; this in turn produced conflict and anxiety to which the child adapted by elaborating "defense mechanisms." The message underlying this formulation was that infants grow up only because they are forced to, with few rewards for doing so.

More modern formulations postulate that pleasure is a welfare emotion that can be experienced not only in the context of satisfying biological needs, but also as a response to mastery of adaptational challenges. Pleasure occurs as part of one's social interaction with others as well as during esthetic experiences. Sandor Rado postulates that the experience of pleasure indicates to the self that it is functioning well; self-esteem is enhanced, thereby increasing the likelihood that adaptational challenges will be successfully met and mastered. Healthy pleasure not only acts as nurturance for the development of self-esteem in this way, but it has a buffer-like effect: a healthy tolerance for pleasure protects the self when it is threatened with pain, decreasing the likelihood of disorganization in the face of that pain.[4] George H. Smith has called pleasure the "fuel of life."[5]

The pleasure associated with adaptational challenges is twofold, namely, that accompanying the activity itself and that associated with the mastery of a particular task. A small child may feel considerable pleasure in the mere act of throwing a ball; pleasure is enhanced if he succeeds in hitting the target. As the child develops, such pleasures are open to considerable influence by parental and social interactions. A child can be made to feel different or "weird" if he has solved a problem using a problem-solving strategy that is different from those used by others; his recreational and occupational interests may differ from those of his parents, who may unwittingly discourage him from pursuing those interests.

How people deal with pleasure appears to have important implications in a wide range of health care problems. A generalized inhibition about pleasure is present in all couples who, present with sexual difficulties and many psychiatric problems as well. When asked the question, "What do you two do to have fun together?" a couple often answers, "Oh, we can't afford to have fun. We're busy paying for our house (or saving up for a new car, etc.)." Pleasure must always he paid for, if it can he experienced at all. It is not something one is allowed to experience in day-to-day living, but rather something one must find outside that arena in alcohol, drugs, or expensive vacations. Some people's "pleasures" must be linked to risk of life or limb as if pleasure and punishment go hand in glove; smoking and mountain climbing are two excellent examples. Other "normal" sources of pleasure become converted into sources of pain. Eating is an activity that most people find enjoyable; for some, however, it is a source of considerable conflict, pain, and suffering. Self-starvation in young people—a means of dealing with complex family conflicts in the area of autonomy—has been elevated to the status of "disease" and given the fancy name "anorexia nervosa." Overeating, the opposite problem, has made obesity one of the major health problems of our age. Alcohol in moderation can be a source of innocent human pleasure; unfortunately, in all too many hands, it leaves a trail of death and destruction in its wake. An individual who "can't handle alcohol" is one who "can't handle pleasure." Compulsive gambling, with its sources in the infantile narcissistic wish to get something for nothing, is often referred to as "a disease."

CHRISTIAN DOCTRINE AND SUFFERING

Since Christianity has contributed so much to our Western notions about pleasure and pain, we should examine the church's teachings about pleasure. These attitudes are summed up neatly by George H. Smith: "Just as Christianity must destroy reason before it can introduce faith, so it must destroy happiness before it can introduce salvation."[6]

Throughout its history, Christianity has been steadfastly not only anti-pleasure but pro-suffering, notwithstanding the gluttonous, licentious, and libidinous behavior of many of its popes and other prelates. The puritan era was simply an extreme manifestation of what amouts to a deep-seated suspicion of pleasure of any sort. While sexual pleasures were the chief source of condemnation, the pleasure inhibition in Christianity was generalized to relate to many other areas. This Christian preoccupation with suffering stems chiefly from Christ's suffering on the cross. As it says in Phil. 2:29, "For unto you it is given in the behalf of Christ, not only to believe on him but also to suffer for his sake." In his epistle to the Romans, Paul wrote, "I beseech you therefore brethren, by the mercies of God, that ye present your bodies a living sacrifice, holy, acceptable unto God, which is your reasonable service" (Rom. 12:1). In his second epistle to the Corinthians, Paul wrote: "Therefore I take pleasure in infirmities, in reproaches, in necessities, in persecutions, in distresses for Christ's sake; for when I am weak, then I am strong" (Cor. 12:10).

Ludwig Feuerbach has pointed out that notwithstanding the claims of its adherents, the Christian religion is one of suffering: "The images of the crucified one which we still see in all churches, represent not the Savior, but only the crucified, the suffering Christ. Even the self-crucifixions among the Christians are, psychologically, a deep-rooted consequence of their religious views. How should not he who has always the image of the crucified one in his mind, at length contract the desire to crucify either himself or another?"[7] The Anglican collect for Holy Saturday could not be more explicit in this regard: "Grant, oh Lord, that as we are baptized into the death of thy blessed Son, our Savior Jesus Christ, so by continually mortifying our corrupt affections we may be buried with him; and that, through the grave, and gate of death, we may pass to our joyful resurrection; for his merits, who died, and was buried, and rose again for us, thy Son Jesus Christ our Lord. Amen."

In Revelations, we learn something about the rewards waiting for the Christians who "suffer for His sake," present their bodies as "a living sacrifice," and take "pleasure in infirmities," continually mortifying their "corrupt affections." Christians are promised that "God shall wipe away all tears from their eyes; and there shall be no more death, nor sorrow, nor crying, neither shall there be anymore pain; for the former things have passed away" (Rev. 21:4).

An offer like this is hard to refuse, and when it is repeated week after week, it should not be suprising to find that the well-programmed Christian has difficulty enjoying the most innocent of pleasures. The nineteenth-century freethinker Robert Ingersoll aptly described the situation: "They [the clergy] must show that misery fits the good for heaven, while happiness prepares the bad for hell; that the wicked get all their good things in this life and the good all their evil; that in this world God punishes the people he loves, and in the next the ones he hates; that happiness makes us bad here, but not in heaven; that pain makes us good here, but not in hell."[8]

At times, the lengths to which Christians have gone to inflict punishment and suffering on themselves in order to curry favor with the divine reaches unbelievable proportions. Historian Rudolph Bell has recently made the startling discovery that the majority of female saints in the Roman Catholic Church were not only severely anorectic (self-starvers), but also addicted to all manner of vicious attacks on their "sinful" bodies. Hair shirts and flagellae were standard equipment. Catherine of Siena's story is fairly typical of the group for whom adequate records exist. She flagellated herself with an iron chain three times daily, each beating lasting one and a half hours with blood running from her shoulders to her feet. Living on bread and water she eventually stopped eating entirely at twenty-five and died at the age of thirty. Catherine reached what must be the nadir of masochism when dressing the purulent cancerous breast sores of a woman she was tending; carefully gathering the pus into a ladle, she drank it all. The antics of the other saints, as reported in Rudolph Bell's book *Holy Anorexia,* are no less bizarre; with role models such as these to guide Christian women through the centuries, we should not be surprised to find an addiction to suffering running through Western society.[9]

If one has been encouraged to suffer in this life in anticipation of the joys of the next, how can one experience true pleasure in the sound of birds singing, a Brahms symphony, or the laughter of children? The dilemma, as posed by Feuerbach, is this: "If God himself suffered for my sake, how can I be joyful, how can I allow myself any gladness, at least on this corrupt earth, which was the theater of his suffering?"[10]

People with a built-in stunting of the capacity to experience pleasure inevitably feel cheated as they go through life, no matter how much they are reminded of the rewards supposedly waiting for them after death. This deep-seated inability to be satisfied by any pleasurable experience keeps alive infantile greed and narcissistic rage, which in turn contributes to deeply disturbed interpersonal relationships and/or psychosomatic illness, or else becomes vented on those who do not share this bizarre belief system.

We live in a society dominated by a religion that promotes suffering as a means of pleasing a narcissistic, capricious deity. At the same time, governments, taxpayers, and insurance companies are all preoccupied with the high costs of health care. In chapter 1 we discussed symptoms of an illness as being determined by an interaction of biological, emotional, and cognitive factors. If an individual has been exposed to the traditional Christian view of suffering (a cognitive, attitudinal factor), it is only natural to expect that this belief will not only affect the symptoms themselves but also the individual's illness behavior. The Christian addiction to suffering must certainly contribute to the illness behavior associated with all types of illness. It is ironic that while health care costs mount, the institution that glorifies suffering for its own sake continues to enjoy the tax-free blessing of the state.

GUILT

Guilt is one of the least understood of the emergency emotions,* but at the same time one of the most destructive. While it may arise spontaneously in the child, its intensity, and its effects on behavior and self-esteem, depend largely on the interaction with parental figures.

Freud viewed guilt as simply fear of the superego (loosely defined as conscience); he considered it to be a normal response to a violation of prohibitions that were instilled in the superego by a loved and feared parental figure. Guilt, according to one modern psychiatric definition, is "an affect associated with self-reproach and need for punishment."[11]

One of the main sources of guilt lies in the infant's response to his own rage when his needs are not satisfied. Initially, he is unable to comprehend what is happening and why. As individuation proceeds and he begins to distinguish himself and his parent as two separate entities, the infant's "thought" processes go something like this: "I am feeling bad (angry)" they (mother and father) must be punishing me by making me feel bad in this way; I cannot be angry at them because they feed me and look after me and I wouldn't

---

*Emergency emotions (fear, rage, and guilt) are those associated with pain or the anticipation of pain; welfare emotions (love, joy, or pride) are those connected with pleasure or the anticipation of pleasure.

want them to punish me more. I must be a 'bad' person for them to want to punish me in this way."

As a child grows, many factors operate to determine what happens to his tendency to reproach himself, i.e., to feel guilty about his anger toward others. Unfortunately, our social attitudes toward anger and its expression encourage parental responses to the child's anger-guilt cycle that reinforce that cycle. Because of their own socialization, parents may be unaware of the potential danger inherent in reinforcing the guilt. Ideally, parents should do what they can to discourage the child from feeling self-punitive when he is angry; instead, all too often they react with some combination of physical punishment and guilt-enhancing responses such as, "Good little boys don't get angry at their mother" or, "Only bad little girls scream like that."

For Christians, guilt is a desirable feeling since it is meant to bring people to Jesus through conversion, confession of sins, and alms-giving. George H. Smith puts it this way: "Guilt, not love, is the fundamental emotion that Christianity seeks to induce—and this is symptomatic of a viciousness in Christianity that few people care to acknowledge."[12]

This prevailing social attitude toward guilt in the Western world has colored theorizing in behavioral science to the point where guilt has been viewed in some quarters as a positive stimulus to sound psychological growth. Carroll Izard, for example, states: "Guilt is the emotion most essential to a development of the affective cognitive structures of conscience and the affective-cognitive-action patterns of moral behavior." He adds that guilt serves as a "check on wanton waste and on sexual and aggressive exploitation."[13] This view, that human beings are frenzied beasts who need to be restrained by making them feel guilty about their impulses, has been voiced so many times from Christian pulpits, it is small wonder that it has influenced people who look at human behavior scientifically. The truth is that human beings want to be able to regulate their impulses in ways that are appropriate to the group, at each stage of life, and such mastery carries with it an increase in self-esteem. Since guilt is never associated with heightened self-esteem, it is difficult to understand how it can contribute to healthy psychological development.

If guilt does have any role to play in promoting psychological growth, it is far outweighed by its destructive role, a point echoed by Franz Alexander: "It is no exaggeration to say that there are no other emotional reactions that play such a permanent and central role in the dynamic explanations of psycho-pathological phenomena as guilt feelings and inferiority feelings."[14]

A number of psychologists have pointed to the destructive impact of guilt-induction. Speaking of the transition from shame to guilt, Erik Erikson has this to say:

The child now feels not only ashamed when found out but also afraid of being found out. He now hears, as it were, God's voice without seeing God. Moreover, he begins automatically to feel guilty even for mere thoughts and for deeds which nobody has watched. This is the cornerstone of morality in the individual sense. But from the point of view of mental health, we must point out that if this great achievement is overburdened by all-too-eager adults, it can be bad for the spirit and for morality itself.[15]

How this process occurs is described by Sandor Rado: "The child is thus forced to move with undue haste from ordinary fear of punishment to fear of conscience, that is, fear of inescapable punishment, and then to guilty fear and the reparative pattern of expiatory self-punishment."[16] Melanie Klein, from the vantage point of her analytic work with children, has pointed out how guilt alienates loved ones from each other: "Feelings of guilt and the drive to make reparation are intimately bound up with the emotion of love. If, however, the early conflict between love and hate has not been satisfactorily dealt with, or if the guilt is too strong, this may lead to a turning away from loved people or even a rejection of them."[17]

Guilt, rather than leading to behavioral change, in fact may reinforce the maladaptive behavior patterns. Parents who use the guilt-inducing "bad boy, bad girl" response may bring the unacceptable behavior to a stop. More often, however, they may produce the opposite effect: the child ends up thinking, "Since I am bad, I will continue until I get enough punishment for being so bad." Many behavioral scientists and criminologists look upon the psychopathic personality as an individual who has no capacity to feel guilt. This is based on the erroneous view that guilt leads to truly adaptive behavior and not simply to seething conformity. In fact, the opposite hypothesis makes more sense, namely, that the propensity of our Christian society to promote the guilt-punishment cycle in individuals is so great that some people become addicted to punishment. This process is behind the phenomenon of scapegoating in families in which one member, usually a child struggling for autonomy, gets attacked and blamed for the family troubles and begins to behave overtly in accordance with his perceived role. Such a child then becomes the "identified patient" in order to protect other members of the family, especially the parents, from having to examine their roles in producing the family distress.

The individual who manifests enough breast-beating, throat-baring behavior may even succeed in getting the rage of his family members converted to sympathy. The contrite alcoholic, compulsive gambler, or wife beater frequently has his destructive maladaptive behavior elevated to the status of a sickness, with the entire health care system becoming involved in changing behavior that he has little desire to alter. On this point, Frieda Fromm-Reichmann says:

In this relationship with authority, the self-punitive acts and experiencing of guilt can be understood as devices for placating the impersonal tyrant. The guilt expressed by the depressive does not carry on to any genuine feeling of regret or effort to change behavior. It is, rather, a means to an end. Merely suffering feelings of guilt is expected to suffice for regaining approval. On the other hand, it may also be seen that achieving a permanent, secure, human relationship with authority is regarded as hopeless. Therefore, no effort to change relationships or to integrate on a better level of behavior is undertaken, and the patient merely resorts to the magic of uttering guilty cries to placate authority.[18]

Leon Salzman makes the same point: "These expressed guilt feelings are often devices to avoid responsibility and to obtain approval through verbalizations rather than action."[19]

In our Western society, the agency most responsible for stimulating and manipulating human guilt is the Christian church. On this point, Guirdham notes: "While many psychiatrists are engaged in trying to free patients from a sense of guilt, a much greater number of priests and ministers are occupied in encouraging its formation."[20] This point is made even more forcefully by philosopher Roger J. Sullivan: "A good deal of preaching is aimed at impressing upon congregations the fact that they are sinners who may not feel as much guilt for their sins as they should."[21]

With the doctrines of Original Sin and Christ's death on the cross to save us from the consequence of our sins, the Christian church gained a vise-like grip on the hearts and minds of its adherents. In order to appreciate how this was possible, it is necessary to understand something about guilt as an interpersonal and political strategy. If A has the power to make B feel guilty, A can control B's behavior by prescribing only those behaviors in B of which A approves. In Christianity, it was not only behavior that was controlled by the stimulation and manipulation of guilt, but the thoughts and fantasies as well. Unclean thoughts were as bad as the deeds themselves; there are frequent references in Paul's letters to keeping the heart pure, which means avoiding even thinking of a prohibited act. In sex relationship therapy, one of the most important tasks is helping people to overcome their guilty fear about sexual fantasies, in order to enable them to experience their sexuality more completely. This guilty fear can be traced to Christian teachings about sexual thoughts.

The Christian church, the House that Guilt Built, behaves very much like the firms that manufacture body soaps and deodorants. The famous Lifebuoy soap ads of the 1930s warned one and all about the dangers of "B.O." (body odor). On the radio, in newspapers and magazines, and even on highway billboards, we were made to feel that our best friends were harboring all kinds of secret thoughts about our smelly bodies. As one ad put it, "Even your best friends won't tell you." However, we could guard against this social sin by the use of Lifebuoy soap, and later on the use of a whole range of deodorants, body sprays, and powders. Since most of these products are aimed at women, we can only assume that the soap industry views women as more smelly than men in the same way that the Christian church has regarded women, from Eve in the Garden through *Malleus Malleficarum*[22] and the witches of Salem, as the major source of temptation for men. The soap industry has literally created a need, and then proceeded to fill that need and their coffers at the same time.

The Christian church created a need for its product by, convincing people that they were basically evil and doomed to hell if they did not accept the Christian world view. The use of human sacrifice to appease angry gods was a feature of many primitive religions and, in some instances, first-born sons were chosen to die. In Christian mythology, the situation is completely reversed. Here God, in order to demonstrate his "love" for us, arranged to have his "only begotten son, in whom I am well pleased," suffer death on the cross in order to save us poor sinful wretches from the clutches of the devil. How a "loving" father could do such a thing to his son, for any reason, baaffled me as a small child; now as a father and grandfather, I am astounded that any sensate human being could be a party to perpetuating such an inhuman myth.

One thing is certain, however. If you believe that someone actually did you a favor of this incredible magnitude (notwithstanding the fact that you did not ask him to do it), your guilt at allegedly pushing the poor fellow to take such an extreme step would be likely to make you feel forever in his debt. In this way, human beings became the pawns of those who claimed to speak in God's name.

Jesus' death on the cross constituted a wonderful "gift" to all humanity from his father, God. The majority of Jews in Israel, however, refused to accept this kind offer and preferred to wait for their own Messiah. For being so ungracious, they became identified as the ones responsible for Jesus' death, and throughout the history of Chistianity have been objects of persecution by Christians, culminating (but not ending) in the Holocaust. Following this decimation of European Jewry by the Nazis, Pope Pius XII proclaimed that the Jews should not be considered Christ killers any longer. It has even become fashionable among Christians to use the bizarre phrase "Judeo-Christian ethics" in an attempt to whitewash the bloody record of Christian injustice toward the Jews.

But if Jesus' sacrifice on the cross was truly an act of redeeming love by God, why should the Jews be persecuted for this, even if they had been responsible for it? Should not they be respected for being agents of such a loving God's will? One can only conclude that down through the ages, the guilt produced in Christians by the sacrifice of Christ on the cross, coupled with the self-loathing stemming from the doctrine of Original Sin, produced so much internal rage that it had to be vented on anyone who did not share their views. And the Jews were the most obvious targets.

CHRISTIAN SELF-SACRIFICE

Christian teaching has always held that Jesus had a number of opportunities to save himself from death, but chose to die on the cross willingly. The glory attached to voluntary martyrdom loomed large in the lives of early Christians. In his letter to the Romans, Paul writes, "Now if we be dead with Christ, we believe that we shall also live with him" (Rom. 6:8). W. H. C. Frend, in his scholarly study of martyrdom in the early Christian church, states: "Death alone for the faith made a Christian a martyr. . . . The Christian's second sealing could not be complete without the, faithful victim's sacrifice by death. But having died 'for the glory of Christ' the martyr had 'fellowship forever with the living God.' "[23]

A. Alvarez's book, *The Savage God*,[24] points out that, contrary to popular myths about throwing the Christians to the lions, often more the Christians made a public nuisance of themselves by willingly jumping into the arena, in the hope of being immediately united with Jesus. But as the church became preoccupied with the task of establishing a terrestrial institution, it responded to this rash of Christian suicides by a series of edicts, culminating in a total ban on such behavior in 693 A.D. at the Council of Toledo. Thus, the "traditional" Christian prohibition against suicide is not traditional at all, but a reaction to the doctrinally supported, deeply rooted suicidal diathesis inherent in the martyrdom of Christ. What happened in Jonestown, Guyana, on the 18th of November, 1978, was simply a rerun of what occurred in Rome during the first few centuries of the Christian era.

Kenneth Wooden's *The Children of Jonestown*[25] points out that, despite the fact that 276 children were included in this "mass suicide," no official investigation was launched by President Carter. Wooden suggests that the friends of Jim Jones in high political office squelched any investigation of this atrocity, which occurred only six weeks before the inauguration of the Year of the Child. An additional reason could be that both President Carter and California governor Jerry Brown—the people most likely to order such an investigation—are Christians. Might they have sensed that such an investigation would force them and the American people as a whole to look into the murky depths of the faith they claim sustains them?

We must acknowledge here that there are different types of suicide. A 65-year-old man facing a prolonged death from untreatable cancer may inject himself with an overdose of a drug in order to spare himself and his family from unnecessary suffering. This case is wholly different from that of the 18-year-old girl who ingests an overdose of her mother's tranquilizers because she is depressed over her boyfriend's rejection. Most of these so-called dyadic suicides, in which someone intends to punish someone else by taking his or her own life, can be traced in large part to the influence of doctrinal Christianity. Just as the church blackmails its followers with the sacrifice of Jesus on the cross, so do suicidal patients try to blackmail loved ones into a state of guilty, abject contrition for the suffering they have "inflicted" on the suicidal victims.

CONCLUSION

We have demonstrated in this chapter that the true Christian has been brainwashed into believing that he was born wicked, that he should suffer as Christ suffered in order to please God, and that he should aspire to a humanly impossible level of perfection. The true Christian should not think well of himself nor attempt to develop supportive human relationships, but put all his trust in God. The church essentially makes people feel guilty for being alive and then professes to protect them from the human "beast" within us all.

But it is in the area of human sexuality and reproduction that we find the Christian church at its Machiavellian best. That is the subject of the next two chapters.

NOTES

1. Jules Henry, *Pathways to Madness* (London: Jonathan Cape, 1972), p. 405.

2. Thomas à Kempis, *The Imitation of Christ* (Chicago: Moody Press, 1980), p. 91.

3. Sigmund Freud, *Beyond the Pleasure Principle,* in James Strachey, trans. and ed., *The Complete Psychological Works of Sigmund Freud* (London: Hogarth Press, 1955), 18: 7–64.

4. Sandor Rado, *Adaptational Psychodynamics* (New York: Science House, 1969), p. 252.

5. George H. Smith. *Atheism: The Case against God* (Buffalo, N.Y.: Prometheus Books, 1979), p. 304.

6. Ibid., p. 308.

7. Ludwig Feuerbach, *The Essence of Christianity,* trans. George Eliot (New York: Harper Torchbooks, 1957), p. 62.

8. Robert G. Ingersoll, "Some Mistakes of Moses," in Gordon Stein, ed., *An Anthology of Atheism and Rationalism* (Buffalo, Prometheus Books, N.Y.: 1980), p. 148.

9. Rudolph M. Bell, *Holy Anorexia* (Chicago: University of Chicago Press, 1985).

10. Feuerbach, *The Essence of Christianity,* p. 62.

11. "Glossary of Psychiatric Terminology," in Alfred M. Freedman, Harold I. Kaplan, and Benjamin J. Sadock, eds., *Comprehensive Textbook of Psychiatry,* 2d ed. (Baltimore, Md.: The Williams and Wilkins Company, 1975), p. 2588.

12. Smith, *Atheism: The Case against God,* p. 304.

13. Carroll Izard, *Human Emotions* (New York: Plenum Press, 1977): pp. 421–25.

14. Franz Alexander, *The Scope of Psychoanlysis* (New York: Basic Books, 1961), p. 129.

15. Erik H. Erikson, "Identity and the Life Cycle," *Psychological Issues* 1, no 1 = Monograph No. 1 (New York: International Universities Press, Inc., 1959), p. 80.

16. Rado, *Adaptational Psychodynamics,* p. 229.

17. Melanie Klein, "Love, Guilt, and Reparation," in John Rickman, ed., *Love, Hate and Reparation. Psychoanalytical Epitomes,* No. 2. (London: Hogarth Press and the Institute of Psychoanalysis), p. 83.

18. Frieda Fromm-Reichmann, *Psychoanalysis and Psychotherapy* (Chicago: University of Chicago Press, 1959), p. 257.

19. Leon Salzman, "Guilt," *Mental Health and Society* 1 (1974): 318.

20. Arthur Guirdham, *Christ and Freud* (London: George Allen and Unwin, Ltd., 1959), p. 97.

21. Roger J. Sullivan, "Psychotherapy: Whatever Became of Original Sin?" in Paul W. Sharky, ed., *Philosophy, Religion and Psychotherapy* (Washington, D.C.: University Press of America, 1982), p. 174.

22. Heinrich Kramer and James Sprenger, *The Malleus Maleficarum* (New York: Dover Publications, 1971).

23. W. H. C. Frend, *Martyrdom and Persecution in the Early Church* (Oxford: Basil Blackwell, 1965), p. 14–15.

24. A. Alvarez, *The Savage God: A Study of Suicide* (New York: Random House, 1972), p. 71.

25. Kenneth Wooden, *The Children of Jonestown* (New York: McGraw-Hill, 1981).

6

Christianity, Sexuality, and Traditional Gender Roles

"The sex drive itself gave organized religion an opportunity to amass what was indisputably the greatest power ever lodged in human hands."
—Rabbi Abraham Feinberg[1]

"Evidently, religious teachings become implicit in the customs and attitudes of a society, eventually regulating both the central tendency of behavior and the expectancy of what people do sexually."
—C. A. Tripp[2]

Sexuality is the source of major problems for many people in Western society. Such issues as sexual dysfunction, pornography, rape, child sexual molestation, unwanted pregnancy, venereal disease, sexual orientation concerns, and AIDS, are persistent preoccupations of the media, the health care profession, and the legal system. Those few health care givers, who are not themselves "eroto-phobic," report that sexual suffering of one form or another can be·found in many of their patients and clients. Behind the divorce rate (nearly one of every three marriages) lurks a lethal combination of sexual and relationship problems. While most people agree that problems with sexuality exist, they are reluctant to explore the origins of the deep-seated attitudes behind these problems. But as long as we avoid tracing these attitudes to their roots, our "solutions" to these problems will continue to be of the band-aid variety.

As in other areas of human existence, our attitudes toward sexuality and sex roles are largely determined by the lessons we learn early in life. Most adults in the English-speaking world would claim that they grew up with no sex education; the truth is that we all grow up with plenty of *sex education,* but very little *sexual enlightenment.*

Education about sexuality is something to which children are constantly exposed, with the lessons usually contained in subtle but repetitive messages. Indeed, it is often said that a parent, a teacher, or a physician cannot help but be a sex educator. One powerful "lesson" is learned every time a parent pushes a child's hand away from the genital area, or insists on referring to the genitals as a "wee wee" or "down there," all the while encouraging the child to learn the correct anatomical terms for all other parts of the body. Another forceful lesson is learned when an obviously embarrassed father tells his son or daughter to "go ask Mother" as a response to the child's first courageous attempt to seek sexual enlightenment. Sexual education occurs when a mother, having failed to prepare her daughter for the menarche, simply tells her to "get a pad from the bathroom," when the terrified girl comes to her mother with sudden unexplained bleeding. Grade school lessons on the human body may bizarrely exclude all mention of the genitals; when examining patients, physicians may ask about the workings of the bladder, lung, and bowel but fail to inquire about sexual functions.

The negative lessons children learn leave them not only sexually ignorant but, worse still, filled with a variety of destructive sexual myths. They become alienated from their sexual natures to a degree that makes it difficult for them to grow up sexually responsive and responsible. Christian teaching about sex makes people vulnerable to all kinds of sexual exploitation: interpersonal, demographic, and commercial.

My colleagues and I at McMaster University in Hamilton, Ontario, have long been concerned with the origins of these sexual attitudes. In a 1981 paper we postulated that such attitudes could be traced to a code of sexual behavior that was and is fundamentally authoritarian, and patently pronatalist in intent.[3] The term "pronatalism" refers to "any attitude or policy that is pro birth, that encourages reproduction, that exalts the role of parenthood."[4] This code is authoritarian as well, in that sexual behaviors are dictated largely by ecclesiastical and/or secular political establishments. Often these pronatalist policies on the part of governments and religious institutions (such as edicts against birth control and abortion) would more properly be termed policies of demographic aggression, since the motive is obviously to enable the "in group" to swamp the "out groups" by sheer weight of numbers. The success of Christian policies of demographic aggression is evidenced by the fact that this religion is now the largest on earth numerically.

Pronatalist attitudes have permeated and shaped Western society to the point where world population growth is, or should be, a source of concern to everyone on the planet. Such attitudes have also penetrated the psyches of Western men and women to the point where they have a profound effect on all aspects of sexuality and reproduction.[5]

This authoritarian pronatalist sex code is characterized by: (1) tolerance, if not actual promotion, of sexual ignorance; (2) proscriptions against sexual awareness in childhood and adolescence; (3) phobic attitudes toward sensual pleasure; (4) prohibition of sexual pleasure over and above that necessary to complete the coital reproductive act; (5) prohibition of sexual behaviors that do not lead to conception (masturbation, oral sex or homosexuality); (6) rejection of individual rights in reproductive regulation; (7) rejection of individual rights in choice of parenthood; (8) downplaying of individual sexual responsibility in favor of rigid adherence to religiously prescribed laws; and (9) gender role stereotyping.

Pronatalism was born in the period of transition between the hunting-gathering stage of social evolution and the agricultural stage, during the so-called neolithic revolution. Hunting-gathering peoples, by the very nature of their lifestyles, were vigorous in their limitation of family size, accomplished largely through infanticide. As anyone who has gone on a hike with small children can appreciate, too many young offspring were a handicap to a nomadic family during the Palaeolithic Age. By contrast, an economy based on agriculture bestows a high economic value even on small children, who can be taught to gather the corn, pull the weeds, herd the cattle, carry food to field hands, and so on. Primitive agricultural people, operating with hunting-gathering emotions about family size, did not change their attitudes readily, and were slow to realize that many children were now an asset and not an encumbrance. The alteration of attitudes about family planning during the Neolithic Age was achieved with the help of primitive religions, largely through the use of fertility worship, in what must have been a truly impressive task of social engineering.

However—and this point is crucial—by the time of the so-called modern religions (Judaism, Hinduism, Christianity, and Islam), there was no longer any need to persist in stressing large families for economic purposes. The motivation to do so now became purely political; modern religious teachings were not designed with the welfare and happiness of the individual in mind.

THE ROLE OF CHRISTIANITY IN FORGING
THE AUTHORITARIAN PRONATALIST SEX CODE

Strategies for promoting large families varied from one religion to another. The Brahmin bride is greeted with this blessing: "May you have eight sons and may your husband live long." In Islam, the practice of polygamy and the Koran's injunction to marry and procreate are two more examples of religion's preoccupation with reproduction. These are what might be called positive pronatalist strategies.

The more negative strategies developed by the Christian church have some of their roots in Judaic law. Following their return from Babylonian exile, the Hebrews passed laws that declared heterosexual intercourse to be the only legal form of sexual expression. Rules about how intercourse was to be conducted were quite specific: "He should have intercourse in the most possible modest manner; he underneath and she above him is considered unchaste." The husband should not "cohabit in the spirit of levity with his wife," and "when having intercourse one should think of matters of the Torah or any holy subject."[6]

The Jewish purity laws involving condemnation of sexual intercourse during the menstrual period are traceable to the fact that a woman cannot get pregnant at that point in her cycle. Psalm 127 gives voice to the Hebrew brand of pronatalism: "As arrows are in the hand of a mighty man, so are children of the youth. Happy is the man that hath his quiver full of them: they shall not be ashamed, but they shall speak with the enemies in the gate." According to the code of Jewish law, "a man is duty bound to take unto himself a wife in order to fulfill the precept of propagation." However, the husband was assumed to have done his duty if he begat a son and daughter, "providing that the son is not a eunuch and the daughter is not incapable of conception."[7] This religious obligation rested on the shoulders of the man, although the bride was blessed with these words: "Our sister, be thou a mother of tens of thousands."[8]

While there are similarities between Jewish and Christian attitudes toward sexuality, the differences are major ones. In spite of the pressure to reproduce in Jewish law, Jews were encouraged to view sexuality as a healthy natural thing to be enjoyed by both husband and wife. In Christianity, sex was regarded as an evil necessity. St. Paul reminds us that because of the wickedness of Eve, presumably in seducing Adam and enjoying the encounter, women were condemned for all eternity: "And Adam was not deceived, but the woman being deceived was in the transgression. Notwithstanding, she shall be saved in childbearing, and if they continue in faith and charity and holiness with sobriety" (2 Tim. 14 and 15). A Jewish man was not supposed to "cohabit with his wife unless it be with her consent" and "it is certainly forbidden to force her."[9] The Christian wife was expected to consent and to perform her sacred duty to such an extent that only in very recent years have secular courts in the Christian West considered the concept of rape within marriage to be a legitmate subject for concern.

Jewish tradition, while similar to the Christian in terms off discouraging noncoital methods of sexual expression, was less vehement in its condemnation of such behavior. Birth control was not mentioned in the code, although nocturnal emissions were certainly frowned upon and were judged to be due to "evil thoughts."[10] The Jewish code required a couple to have only two children, provided each child was capable of procreating in turn. Christian tradition encouraged large families, even though, as John T. Noonan, Jr., has pointed out, this was not an explicit aspect of doctrine.[11] The Christian church, building on its Jewish foundations, borrowed freely from other religions, developed many of its own teachings, and inexorably harnassed the sexuality of its followers to serve its policies of demographic aggression. It had no need to show its hand by being explicit about its aims.

What is remarkable about Christian attitudes toward sexuality and repro-duction, is the complete absence of any reference to them in the teachings of Jesus that have come down to us. It is quite possible that, given the tenor of many of the other teachings attributed to Jesus, he did say something about this very important aspect of human life. It may even be that Jesus' words were expunged from the record, simply because his ideas did not square with the doctrines being promulgated so energetically by the early church fathers. As Reay Tannahill has put it, "It is undoubtedly a tribute (if an ambigous one) to such men as St. Jerome and St. Augustine that much of what the modern world still understands by 'sin' stems not from the teachings of Jesus of Nazareth, or from the tablets handed down from Sinai, but from the early sexual vicissitudes of a handful of men who lived in the twilight days of Imperial Rome."[12]

In the decades following Jesus' death on the cross and "resurrection," his followers were not preoccupied with such mundane matters as rules of sexual and reproductive behavior, since they were waiting for the Master's return. But when Jesus' disciples realized that the second coming was not imminent, they set about the task of developing an earthly institution in his name. Again to quote Tannahill, "propagation of the faithful was a useful aid to propagation of the faith, and the church resigned itself to having its flock regularly augmented by new lambs."[13]

A tradition of asceticism stemming from long years of waiting formed the foundation on which the sexual philosophy was built. It might be said that the early church's reverence for chastity, still (theoretically) preserved in the clergy and religious orders of the Roman Catholic Church, gradually gave way to a reluctant sanction of sexual intercourse within marriage, while at the same time forbidding all other forms of sexual expression that could not lead to conception. In the early years of the church, a variety of institutionalized attitudes about sex and reproduction affected the development of Christian doctrine, both positively and negatively. The Gnostics believed in a strict dualism and saw the true believer as someone who rejected the evil material world completely in order to embrace the holy realm of the spiritual. Most Gnostics lived ascetic lives, rejecting reproduction, if not sexuality itself. Gnosticism represented a powerful segment of the Christian community awaiting Jesus' return; when the need to make a home on earth became obvious, Gnostic views on reproduction had to be supplanted. Gnosticism became, in essence, one of the first heresies to be stamped out by the Christian church; but in stamping out Gnosticism, as Vern Bullough has stated, "the early Christian Church came to be deeply influenced by it, and in the long run its attitudes toward sex seem to have been more influenced by the ascetic Gnostics than the more earthly Jews."[14]

In his book *Contraception,* John T. Noonan, Jr., traces some of the origins of the church's doctrines on sexuality and reproduction to the Stoic philosophers, whose ideas were "very much in the air the intellectual converts to Christianity breathed," and who "had a powerful grip on the minds of many of the ablest Christians."[15] The Stoical approach to sexuality was concerned with control of all bodily desires, the watchwords being "nature, virtue, decorum, and freedom from excess." For the Stoic, passion in any form, even in the marriage bed, was frowned on; sexual intercourse was for procreation only. The Stoics were also partial to "rational self-sufficiency," a goal which, as Noonan pointed out in what must be the understatement of the century, the Christian intellectuals did not adopt.

Christian doctrine, to the effect that sex was for reproduction only, received a strong impetus from the teachings of St. Augustine. Augustine had been a member of a heretical sect called the Manichees, who were followers of a third-century prophet Mani. Manichaeism bore a strong resemblance to the ascetic Gnosticism of the first and second centuries, especially in its rejection of procreation. In his eleven years as a disciple of Mani, Augustine had never been able to climb to the highest rank of the order because of his strong sexual appetites. When he became a convert to orthodox Christianity, Augustine succeeded in curbing those appetites; his subsequent teachings contributed to the strengthening of the church's iron grip on the uteri of female Christians for centuries.

Sixteen hundred years of indoctrination by Christian teachings on human sexuality and reproduction constitute the basis for the authoritarian pronatalist sex code that has devastated the sexual and reproductive lives of so many human beings in the Western world. Forged in the infancy of Christianity, preoccupied with producing ever more Christians in the struggle against non-Christians, this code has been used and manipulated by many secular states in order to further policies of military aggression, economic aggrandizement, and colonial expansion.

Christian apologists have always denied that the church's teaching on sex and reproduction constituted a strategy to swamp other religions by the sheer weight of numbers. However, in 1984, Pope John Paul II let the cat out of the bag when, shortly before his triumphal tour of Canada, he criticized Catholics for the manner in which they were using the church-approved "natural" method of family planning. This is the technique colloquially known as "Vatican roulette," by which abstention from intercourse during the woman's fertile period is acceptable to the church as a means of regulating reproductivity. An attempt by some Roman Catholic physicians to cloak this method in medical responsibility by using the woman's body temperature as a guide to ascertaining the safe period has led to the use of the quaint neologism, "sympto-thermic" method of birth control.

The pope complained to those few Catholics still faithful to the spirit of *Humanae Vitae* and still using the rhythm method: "The use of infertile periods in married life can become a source of abuses if the couples seek in such a way to avoid *without just reasons* procreation, lowering procreation below the *morally correct level of births* for their family (my italics)."[16] This demographic paranoia on the part of John Paul is strangely reminiscent of the words of Adolph Hitler who wrote in *Mein Kampf*, "Anyone who wants to secure the existence of the German people by a self-limitation of its reproduction, is robbing it of its future."[17] Hitler was as much in opposition to contraception and abortion as is John Paul II. By his statement, the pope made it clear that morality was attached not to the *method* of birth control, but to the *number of births it prevented.* In spite of the pope's concern, it is well known that the "natural" method of birth control is not an effective means of contraception, even in the hands of highly motivated, devout Catholic couples. Hence couples relying on this method are likely to have more babies than those who use one of the more effective methods prohibited by *Humanae Vitae.* The church does not stop to consider whether such babies are welcomed by their parents.

It is worth examining in detail the elements of the pronatalist sex, code in order to demonstrate how each operates to maximize the number of births.

TOLERANCE, IF NOT ACTUAL PROMOTION, OF SEXUAL IGNORANCE

A pronatalist sex code favors sexual ignorance for a very obvious reason: the more ignorant people are about sexuality and reproduction, the less power they have to regulate that reproductivity. Nature takes its own course.

The role of Christianity in continuing this state of affairs should be obvious to anyone with even a rudimentary knowledge of the state of sexual education in our society. Christian clerics and lay militants are in the forefront of opposition to the implementation of sex education in the schools. Their argument is that learning about sex will stimulate young people to get involved in sexual activity before they are married, notwithstanding the fact that learning about nutrition and the human gastrointestinal system does not make people suddenly want to eat. In fact, the opposite is more likely to be the case. A great deal of early sexual adolescent activity can be traced to teenagers' attempts to learn by doing, often with disastrous consequences. The available scientific evidence indicates that sexual enlightenment tends to cause adolescents to indulge in sexual intercourse much later than nonenlightened adolescents, although the former may be involved in noncoital sexual behavior. When passion overrides the effects of the preaching, the unenlightened adolescent, steeped in the pronatalist myth that sex equals intercourse, is programmed to reject noncoital sexual activities in favor of unprotected coitus.

Australian researchers Ronald and Juliette Goldman attempted to determine the extent of childhood sexual knowledge by studying over 800 children, aged five, seven, nine, eleven, and fifteen, in four parts of the world: Sweden, England, Australia, and North America (specifically the Buffalo area of upstate New York and St. Catherines in nearby Ontario, Canada).[18] The Goldmans administered to the children a number of age-specific questions based on the developmental theories of Jean Piaget and Lawrence Kohlberg. They discovered that Swedish children showed a much earlier comprehension of the origin of babies and the biological role of parents than did the children in all the English-speaking countries. Twenty percent of all English-speaking parents refused permission for their children to be involved in the study compared to only 5 percent of the Swedish parents. One explanation for this is that although until recently the Lutheran Church was the state church in Sweden, in fact Christianity came late to Scandinavia and its doctrines penetrated Swedish society and the Swedish personality to a lesser depth than in the English-speaking world. Sweden has developed probably the best sex education programs in the world thus far. According to the Goldman study, North American children appear to have the least and longest-delayed sex education of all the four areas studied.

The socialization process that results in so much ignorance also tends to produce attitudes toward erotic issues that are actually phobic. William Fisher and his colleagues, who developed an erotophobic-erotophilic scale, have demonstrated that negative attitudes toward sexuality make it difficult for people to assimilate information about this aspect of life. This body of research has also demonstrated that erotophobic people tend to be very authoritarian in outlook and to adhere to very traditional gender or sex roles. Erotophobia among both males and females is associated with both poor contraceptive usage and, as might be expected, considerable sexual dysfunction.[19]

A common argument used by physicians and other health care workers to justify their avoidance of the subject of sex with patients and clients, is the fear of imposing a particular set of beliefs on a vulnerable individual. They fail to see that by this very act of avoidance, they are clearly promoting a belief system that has been demonstrated to produce untold human misery.

THE PROSCRIPTION AGAINST SEXUAL AWARENESS IN CHILDHOOD AND ADOLESCENCE

Hand in hand with society's promotion of sexual ignorance in children is the attempt to prevent children from recognizing that they are sexual beings themselves, and that they have feelings and bodily responses that constitute the beginnings of adult sexuality.

That children will be harmed if they became aware of their own and others' sexuality is a belief that runs deep in our society. Children are still punished for masturbating or exploring their own bodies in a potentially pleasurable way, as well as for indulging in sex play with a, friend of either sex.

In his *Three Essays on the Theory of Sexuality,* published in 1908, Sigmund Freud flew in the face of the authoritarian pronatalist sex code by asserting that children were indeed sexual beings. The response to these essays is described by Freud's biographer, Ernest Jones: "The book certainly brought down on him more odium than any other of his writings. *The Interpretation of Dreams* had been hailed as fantastic and ridiculous, but the *Three Essays* were shockingly wicked. Freud was a man with an evil and obscene mind. . . . This assault on the pristine innocence of childhood was unforgiveable."[20]

One particularly destructive myth is that by deliberately keeping children in ignorance about sexuality, we are "protecting" them from something. The truth is quite the opposite. It is this very ignorance and socially sanctioned lack of understanding that contributes to the sexual victimization of children by adults. If a child's healthy natural curiosity is frustrated by parents and teachers, we should not be surprised that this thwarted curosity constitutes some of the motivation to go along with the favorite uncle, father, or family friend when he makes inappropriate advances. Stevi Jackson's *Childhood and Sexuality* echoes these sentiments: "We do more harm than good in enforcing sexual ignorance on children. In attempting to protect children from sex, we expose them to danger; in trying to preserve their innocence, we expose them to guilt."[21]

PHOBIC ATTITUDES TOWARD SENSUAL PLEASURE

A couple had twins, a boy and a girl. On visits to the husband's family when the babies were a few months old, their father hugged and kissed each of them equally. His Baptist relatives were alarmed at his behavior with his infant son and warned that the boy might grow up to become a "sissy" or a "homosexual" if the father persisted in this affectionately sensuous behavior. Shere Hite, in her report on male sexuality, found that most of the men surveyed had wanted, but not had, a relationship with their fathers that was open and honest, but above all one that was physically affectionate. Their views were expressed by one man who said, "If only I had had a warm, loving, physically affectionate man for a father. The father should not be afraid to touch and cuddle his son."[22]

One common situation between couples with sexual problems is a male who resists being sensuous with his female partner. Such behaviors as cuddling and caressing are not part of his repertoire (often to the dismay of the woman), simply because he does not feel he "needs it." By this the man means that he is able to obtain an erection for intercourse and, given the fixation on coitus that is part of the sexual socialization of males, he is unable to see the need for further sensuous pleasures. Such men are unable to hear it when their wives state that this form of sexual pleasure is important to them, so fixed are they on coitus and their own coital performance. While males in our society tend to deny their needs for sensuousness in their sexual relationships, such needs do exist. One cogent piece of evidence is the existence of massage parlors, in which males can indulge in sensuous pleasure dissociated from their sexual relationships; such pleasure can be enjoyed not only anonymously, but also with a degree of passivity that would be unthinkable for men to negotiate in their sexual relationships with their partners.

In chapter 4, the importance of skin-to-skin contact for the healthy development of the infant was stressed. Fairly persuasive evidence exists of a correlation between the somatosensory deprivation of infants and the predilection to violence. In his study of the possible relationship between these two factors,[23] neuropsychologist James W. Prescott has compared a culture's tolerance of, or affinity for, violence and its attitudes to infant physical affection and to premarital sexual activity. The least violent societies were those that provided a great deal of infant physical somatosensory affection and manifested a high degree of tolerance for adolescent sexual activity. The most violent societies were those that provided infants with minimal physical affection and did not tolerate teenage sex. Prescott also found that those societies providing the greatest amount of physical affection were also characterized by low rates of theft, minimal physical punishment of children, and low religious activity.

Prescott's comparative study also revealed that some cultures with a high level of infant somatosensory affection and stimulation also exercised a very punitive attitude toward adolescent premarital sexual activity; these cultures tended to be more violent than those that were tolerant of adolescent premarital sexual behavior, whether or not infants were provided with plenty of somatosensory stimulation. For Prescott, "The detrimental effects of infant physical affectional deprivation seem to be compensated for later in life by sexual body pleasure experiences during adolescence."[24]

The phobia about sensuousness serves the goals of pronatalism by blocking all the potentially pleasurable sexual sideroads on the way to the "real thing"—

coitus. The Christian rejection of pleasure that pervades our society, coupled with Christianity's fanatically coercive heterosexuality, reinforces that phobia. Prescott's study demonstrates that such a collection of attitudes predisposes a society to violence. And when it comes to violence, our Western Christian society has been among the leaders of the pack. Onward, Christian soldiers!

THE PROHIBITION OF SEXUAL PLEASURE
BEYOND IMPREGNATION

Basic Christian doctrine regarding sexuality had no room for pleasure. St. Paul summed it up when he said, "Better to marry than to burn [with desire]" (1 Cor. 7:9). The message one gets from Christian doctrine is that it would be better if folks got along without sex, except that this is the only way to create more Christians to fulfill the church's aim of swamping demographically those non-Christians who refuse to convert to the one true faith.

Men were the only ones meant to have any physical enjoyment from their sexuality, but only enough to enable them to "perform" their duty of sexual intercourse; sexual pleasure for its own sake (not in the service of reproduction) was frowned on. Women were not expected to experience plea-sure at all except in the knowledge that they were pleasing their husbands in their role as mothers.

Paradoxically, even though women were not meant to enjoy lovemaking, they were made to feel that they were responsible for arousing the sexuality of males, who in turn were made to feel so guilty for the small amount of pleasure they got from sexual intercourse that they had to project the blame onto women. The infamous *Malleus Maleficarum* (*The Witch's Hammer*), written by two Dominican priests, James Sprenger and Heinrich Kramer,[25] and published in 1486, laid the blame for "carnal" impulses squarely on the shoulders of women, who were often burned at the stake as witches if they showed any overt evidence of having sexual impulses: "'All witchcraft comes from carnal lust, which is in women insatiable."[26] The book was endorsed by the church, accepted in every country in Europe, and over the next two hundred and fifty years went through more than thirty editions.[27] It is little wonder that it took another two hundred years before women began to feel secure enough to come out from under the threat of being burned at the stake if they acknowledged sexual feelings openly.

A prevailing myth is that women have sexual problems more than men, and indeed in sex therapy clinics many more women than men are the identified patients. However, complementing the problem of many of these sexually dysfunctional women are male partners who, although "functional" in terms of the pronatalist sex code, in reality show a great deal of limitation in their ability to experience pleasure. These men are often totally unable to tolerate the closeness and intimacy with their partners that constitutes the source of much of the pleasure in a healthy sexual relationship.

Another common myth regarding male sexuality is that if a man "wants it all the time" or "has to have it every night or three times a day," he is a highly sexed individual. And in these instances, it is often the man's female partner who presents as "pathological," complaining of a "lack of sexual desire" or an inability to achieve orgasm. In reality, the male is often a sexual cripple, with a capacity for sexual pleasure so limited that he can only tolerate frequent physiological orgasms coitally produced. Unable to enjoy a fully satisfying sexual experience with a partner, he simply uses his partner's vagina as a substitute for his hand to relieve the physiological tension, like a nibbler at a sumptuous banquet. It is common for the male partner of such a sexually "dysfunctional" female to state after a course of therapy for "her" problem that he did not realize how much he had been missing.

THE PROHIBITION OF SEXUAL BEHAVIORS NOT LEADING TO CONCEPTION

Masturbation

In devising a code of sexual behavior that would guarantee the survival of the church, the early fathers left no stone unturned in their determinations to convert the female uterus into a factory for turning out Christian babies. Since masturbation is the simplest form of sexual gratification, and requires no partner, special condemnation was reserved for it. According to Tannahill, the West's Christian society is the only one in which masturbation was totally proscribed.[28]

In Matt. 5:30, Jesus says: "And if thy right hand offend thee cut it off, and cast it from thee: for it is profitable for thee that one of thy members should perish, and not that thy whole body should be cast into hell." Whether Jesus was referring to genital self-stimulation has been the subject of considerable debate. However, in seeking scriptural authority for its teachings on masturbation, the church has relied heavily on the story of Onan, whose "sin" was not masturbation but rather *coitus interruptus*. In the Genesis story, Er, the son of Juda, married Tamar and shortly afterward offended God and was promptly killed. By terms of the Hebrew Levirate (brother-in-law) marriage, Onan, brother of Er, was expected to marry and impregnate Tamar in order that his dead brother would have progeny. Onan, resenting the fact that any child he fathered would not be his, "spilled his seed upon the ground," *not* inside the womb of his new wife. The word onanism, applied to masturbation, was first used in the eighteenth century. In 1710, an ex-clergyman turned quack published *Onania, or the heinous sin of self-pollution and all its frightful consequences in both sexes, considered with physical and spiritual advice.* The author, whose name was Bekker, by this misunderstanding of the story of Onan, introduced a term into the language that would remain for two centuries. His book went through eighty editions and was translated into several languages.[29] In 1760, a respected Swiss physician named Tussot published *Onanism, or a treatise upon the disorders produced by masturbation,* in which he claimed that masturbation was not only a sin and a crime but was directly responsible for a multitude of afflictions from "consumption" to "insanity." Benjamin Rush, the father of American psychiatry, and Henry Maudsley, the nineteenth-century British psychiatrist who gave his name to the world-famous psychiatric institute in London, added the weight of their authority to the irrational panic over masturbation. "Masturbatory insanity" was, according to Maudsley, "characterized by extreme perversion of feeling and corresponding derangement of thought, in earlier stages, and later by failure of intelligence, nocturnal hallucinations, and suicidal and homicidal propensities."[30] Twentieth-century admonitions about failing eyesight and hair on the palms seem mild by comparison.

Self-pleasuring violates more than one of the doctrines of Christianity. First, the individual is preoccupied with his or her own self, and that in itself runs counter to church teachings. Second, he or she is preoccupied with pleasure, and all earthly pleasures are suspect. Third, he or she is concerned with pleasures of the "flesh," which were open to condemnation from the time of St. Paul, who was constantly warning his followers throughout the church to "abstain from fleshly lusts which war against the soul" (Pet. 2:11). Finally, masturbation is a nonprocreative sex act. Small wonder, then, that the Christian teaching regarding masturbation has contributed and continues to contribute to so much human suffering. In 1975, the Vatican reaffirmed that masturbation was "an intrinsically and seriously disordered act," all the while acknowledging that modern psychological and sociological evidence showed it to be a normal aspect of human sexual development and behavior.[31] Don't bother me with facts, my mind is made up!

One of the most revealing "findings" of the Goldman and Goldman study, cited earlier, was not a finding at all but rather an artifact of the study design. In pretesting the sexual vocabulary to be used in the questionnaire, the authors eliminated some words that, in their judgment, "transgressed what might be acceptable to parents." Among these were words relating to homosexuality and masturbation, the latter causing such embarrassment in the trial interviews that it had to be excluded. The authors correctly termed this a "sad indication in itself of the state of communication about sexuality."[32]

Homosexuality

The word "homosexual," which was imported into English from German by the psychologist Havelock Ellis in 1897,[33] has always been surrounded by considerable confusion as to whether it was an adjective applied to a sexual act between two people of the same gender or a noun referring to an individual who performed such sexual acts exclusively. If it is a noun, at what point in the Kinsey scale of homosexuality does it apply? Some semantic confusion has been swept away by the use of the word "gay" to denote individuals who are exclusively homosexual in their orientation and behavior, reserving the adjective "homosexual" to apply to sexual acts.

Early fertility cults, perhaps even very ancient tribes of Israel, had incorporated in their religious ceremonies a variety of ritualized sexual behaviors involving priests, priestesses, and worshipers. Male-to-male fellatio was only one of these ritualized activities, one that still survives in at least one primitive culture.[34] The practice gradually died out, no doubt because of a growing concern about all forms of nonprocreative sexual behavior in agricultural societies, and was eventually contained within territories with boundaries that had to be protected against intruders.

The condemnation of homosexual behavior is explicit in Lev. 18:22: "Thou shalt not lie with mankind as with womankind; it is abomination." In Lev. 20:13, the prohibition is put in stronger terms: "If a man also lie with mankind, as he lieth with a woman, both of them have committed an abomination: they shall surely be put to death: their blood shall be upon them." Philo, a Hebrew philosopher writing at the time of Jesus, uses an agricultural metaphor to express his distaste of homosexuality. "Like a bad husbandman," the homosexual "spends his labor night and day on soil from which no growth at all can be expected."[35]

Although Jesus has nothing to say in the gospels to indicate his own views either for or against homosexuality, St. Paul made no bones about declaring how he felt on the subject. In Rom. 1:27 he states, "And likewise also the men, leaving the natural use of the woman, burned in their lust one toward another; men with men working that which is unseemly, and receiving in themselves that recompense of their error which was meet." In Cor. 6:9, Paul warns again that "abusers of themselves with mankind" shall not inherit the kingdom of God.

In third-century Rome, before Christianity became the state religion, laws were passed making homosexuality punishable by death. By this time, the Roman state had become very anxious about its declining birth rate and was undoubtedly influenced by the rise of Christianity, whose attitudes about reproduction were so blatantly pronatalist. When Christianity did assume political power in the West, the lot of the homosexual was not a happy one.

As late as the sixteenth century in England, laws were passed making homo-sexual acts punishable by death. Nineteenth-century England, as aggressively pronatalist as any state in history, saw the famous prosecution of Oscar Wilde for "the sin that dares not speak its name." Nazi Germany persecuted and killed gays for the same reason that England persecuted them in the nineteenth century: gays cannot produce more Englishmen or more Germans.

Historian John Boswell has reexamined the record of the church's doc-trines concerning homosexuality and its treatment of homosexuals.[36] While he acknowledges that the Christian establishment mistreated homosexuals, he tries to explain away the doctrinal support for such behavior, insisting that the persecution of homosexuals originates in something other than church doctrine. To support his view Boswell cites numerous instances throughout the life of the church in which male-to-male homosexuality was openly tolerated, even among priests and monks. His argument about the lack of doctrinal support is not very convincing, however.

The inconsistency of responses on the part of the Christian establishment, secular and ecclesiastical, to homosexuality, as well as to other forms of non-procreative sexuality, is more open to explanations having to do with the state of that establishment's demographic "health." Demographic anxiety exists when a more populous neighboring state shows signs of becoming unfriendly, at which time we are likely to see negative reactions to nonprocreative sexuality and abortion. Given the political conditions facing the Jews before Christ, it is small wonder that they developed pronatalist attitudes toward sexuality. Similarly, the early Christian church was eager to expand and hence formulated negatives doctrines concerning masturbation, homosexuality, birth control, and abortion that coerced people to reproduce. By the time the church reached what has been termed the "zenith of the medieval papacy"[37] around 1100 and felt its power to be secure, it relaxed its severe pronatalist pressures. The position on abortion was mollified as the doctrine of delayed ensoulment* came more to the fore, making it possible for early abortions to be performed licitly.[38] Boswell points out that this was also a period of an "extraordinary flower-ing of gay love," especially among the clergy of the day, although there were others in the church who urged the strongest of sanctions against gay priests.[39]

Birth Control

The most vivid memory of my psychiatric training is also a very sad one. It concerns a visit to the crèche† at a Roman Catholic hospital in Montreal

---

*The doctrines of immediate and delayed ensoulment will be discussed in the section, "Abortion."

†The holding place for unwanted infants waiting for adoption or until they were old enough to be transferred to an orphanage.

in 1960. Through the glass we saw what seemed to be a veritable sea of white cribs containing tiny figures, some of them sleeping, but most of them sitting up, completely motionless and staring at us through the glass with empty, lifeless eyes. There was one exception. Near the nurses' station was a plump black baby of about ten months, standing up in his crib, smiling and moving about playfully. As we approached him, he engaged us with his eyes and was obviously trying to involve us in some kind of interaction through the glass. We were all puzzled by the sharp contrast between this obviously healthy, vibrant little boy and the almost marasmic infants around him.

We did not have to ponder this question long. Soon it was time for the nurses to change shift, and as each nurse left the floor, she walked over to the black baby and said goodbye to him, some hugging him, others chucking him under the chin and laughing with him. As each new nurse came on duty, this process was repeated. The other infants were all but ignored. The nurses, all white, had singled out the one black child in the crèche as a kind of pet and he was thriving on it. In this instance, it was good to be black. This experience convinced me of two things. The first was the appalling effect of maternal deprivation. Second, as I looked at all these unwanted children, I became convinced that the teachings of the Christian church about contraception and abortion, at that time reflected in the laws of the land, were unquestionably immoral. This experience took place almost a decade before the Canadian Criminal Code was amended (over strident objections from many Christian clergy) to make the sale of contraceptives legal and to legalize abortions under certain circumstances.

Although, according to the book of Genesis, "God" advised his creatures to "increase and multiply; fill the earth and subdue it" (Gen. 1:27-28), there is no evidence of a strong proscription of the use of contraception in Jewish religious tradition. The promotion of births relied more on exhortation than on the strict regimentation of the sexual life that became part of Christian teaching. In Jewish law, "conjugal duty" on the part of males was recommended on the basis of occupation: for men of independent means, once every day; for laborers, twice a week; for ass drivers, once a week; for camel drivers, once in thirty days; and for sailors, once in six months.[40] By the beginning of the Christian era, the more relaxed Jewish attitude toward sexuality gave way to something approaching the orthodox Christian concept. Philo promoted the idea that sexual intercourse was for procreation only, and hinted that God would punish those who had intercourse for pleasure.[41]

While the New Testament contains many passages, especially in the letters of Paul, indicating the specifically procreative role of sexual relations, it says nothing specific about contraception itself. Later church teachings about contraception were developed as part of an overall strategy of placing Christians on a reproductive assembly line.

In his writings on sex and marriage, St. Augustine, the libertine turned ascetic, sums up the approach that had been gradually developed in the first four centuries of the the church: "What is unlawful food in the wantonness of the belly and gullet, this is unlawful intercourse seeking in lust no offspring."[42] This injunction was put in even stronger terms by the Bishop of Arles in the sixth century:

> Who is he that cannot warn that no woman may take a potion so that she is unable to conceive or condemns in herself a nature which God willed to be fecund. As often as she could have conceived or given birth, of that many homicides she will be held guilty, and, unless she undergoes suitable penance, she will be damned by eternal death in hell.[43]

In the fifteenth century, the *Malleus Maleficarum* uses similar language: "And note, further, that the Canon speaks of loose lovers who, to save their mistresses from shame, use contraceptives, such as potions, or herbs that contravene nature, without any help from devils. And such penitents are to be punished as homicides."[44]

The teachings of the Christian church on birth control became deeply embedded in the social and political fabric of the Western world. Because Christian doctrine had laid the groundwork, secular states had no difficulty passing laws against birth control in order to satisfy their pronatalist ambitions or to allay their demographic anxieties. All too often, God's name was invoked to justify such laws in nineteenth-century England, and in the United States and Nazi Germany in the twentieth century. And just as politicians were able to hide their aggressive intentions behind Christian doctrine, so were physicians able to cloak their inhumane treatment of women behind the same set of teachings. Until well into the present century, many physicians were preaching against birth control on the basis that it was harmful to women's health as well as against the laws of the deity—the same arguments being used by some physicians today in connection with abortion, without a shred of scientific evidence. The birth control battle was originally waged by people outside the medical profession, many of them women, notably Margaret Sanger in the United States and Marie Stopes in England. And it is no accident that the first book on the medical aspects of contraception in this century was written not by a physician but by a sociologist.[45]

Most people remain unaware of how recent the birth control movement really is. It was in 1912 that the president of the American Medical Association urged physicians to get involved in the birth control issue, a move that provoked a great deal of controversy but within and outside the profession. And not until 1932 did the Church of England give a very cautious approval of artificial birth control, which also brought forth a great deal of medical condemnation.

In violation of the Canadian Criminal Code, Dorothea Palmer started a birth control center in Ottawa in the early 1930s and distributed birth control pamphlets. In 1936, she was charged and tried after she responded to a request from a Catholic mother for contraceptive advice. At her trial in Eastview, near Ottawa, Palmer was acquitted and the Crown's appeal was rejected by the Appeal court. However, the Criminal Code provisions under which she had been charged were not changed until 1969.[46]

Although most Protestant denominations do not now actively forbid the use of contraceptives, the Roman Catholic church officially still does so, in spite of the fact that the majority report of the Birth Control Commission in the 1960s recommended the change in the church's position. The progressive voice in the Vatican was stilled in the late 1970s following the untimely death of Pope John Paul I, who favored artificial forms of birth control.[47]

Abortion

In line with its determination to exert rigid control over the reproductive apparatuses of its followers, from the second century on, the early church fathers made abortion as serious a sin as infanticide. The basis of the prohibition was the doctrine of immediate ensoulment, which stated that since the soul entered the body at conception, the life of the unbaptized fetus could not be taken. Baptism was the key. But while abortion of the ensouled fetus was a sin, it was apparently all right many centuries later for Spaniards to baptize infant Indian babies in the Americas, then dash their brains out so that they could go to heaven before they had an opportunity to commit sin.[48] The competing doctrine of delayed ensoulment held that the soul entered the female embryo at eighty days and the male at forty days. The gender difference had to do with the phallic tubercle in the embryo, the forerunner of the penis, which appears at forty days gestation. If no tubercle appeared by eighty days gestation, God presumably gave the embryo a female soul.

The doctrine of immediate ensoulment prevailed during the early centuries of the church as it struggled to dominate Europe; by the Middle Ages, when the church felt secure, the doctrine of delayed ensoulment prevailed. In the thirteenth century, Pope Innocent III wrote a letter to a monk who had impregnated his mistress, in which the pope advised him that it was not "irregular" to abort the fetus if it was not yet vivified, i.e., ensouled.[49] In the Roman Catholic church, this relaxed attitude toward abortion more or less continued until 1869, when Pope Pius IX proclaimed, in Constitution *Apostolicae Sedis,* that the distinction between the formed (ensouled) and unformed fetus was no longer valid; the soul entered the body at conception. Henceforth abortion at any stage of gestation could result in excommunication.

This volte-face is explainable in terms of the same demographic factors that motivated other aspects of the church's doctrinal treatment of sexuality and reproductivity. In 1869, the Vatican was engaged in a life-and-death military struggle with the forces of Italian nationalism; Pius's armies had lost control of the papal states, which in 1848 had comprised one-third of the Italian peninsula. By 1869, the pope was left with what is now Vatican City. The pope, transformed from a liberal to a bitter reactionary almost overnight, after having lost so much temporal power, moved to strengthen his spiritual control over Catholics everywhere. Pius followed the edict against abortion by convening the first Vatican council in 1870, at which the dogma of papal infallibility was proclaimed, much to the consternation of many of the bishops present.

Similar demographic political factors lie behind the enactment of every secular anti-abortion law. The first English law against abortion was enacted in 1803, common law prior to that date having held that abortion before quickening (the point when the woman first feels fetal movement) was not illegal. In 1801, England had conducted its first census and discovered that its population was less than half that of France, with whom she had been at war intermittently since 1793, and whom she would continue to fight until the Battle of Waterloo in 1815. In the brief lull in hostilities in 1803, Britain was in a vulnerable position, similar to the one she faced in 1940 against Nazi Germany. It was in the climate generated by England's precarious military situation, then, that the first anti-abortion law was passed. This was followed by more stringent anti-abortion legislation in 1828, 1837, and 1861, as Britain attempted to swamp the French demographically in Canada and the Irish in Ireland, and to provide a never-ending flow of workers for her factories at home and soldiers to defend her growing empire overseas. In the United States, the first anti-abortion law was passed in Connecticut in 1822, stemming from that state's concerns over its loss of population westward. Other states soon followed suit as the westward migration swelled, displacing native populations with European immigrants, whose higher birthrates were causes of grave concern among the native American politicians and citizenry.

In Germany in the early 1930s, a campaign to liberalize abortion laws was nipped in the bud when the Nazis came to power; these worthies made abortion a crime punishable by death. In the early 1920s, Russia had liberalized its abortion laws, primarily to free up women for the labor force. But in 1936, influenced by events in Germany, the Soviet government suddenly reversed its position and declared all abortions illegal. This example of demographic panic proved more of a hindrance than a help when Hitler finally invaded Russia in 1941; the children born in the interim to women who might formerly have sought an abortion were all under four years old. Russia's abortion laws were again liberalized in 1955.

I have documented the struggle to liberate women from the burden of compulsory pregnancy in an earlier publication, *Compulsory Parenthood;* in the interests of completeness, however, I shall summarize that struggle here.

Sweden, along with other Scandinavian countries, led the way in liberalizing abortion laws; by 1975, that country passed a law not only making abortion in the first twelve weeks simply a matter for the woman to decide, but laying the burden of justification for refusing an abortion squarely on the shoulders of the physician. In the United States, decades of battling against the old anti-abortion laws by feminist groups and others opposed to compulsory pregnancy led to the famed Supreme Court *Roe* v. *Wade* decision in 1973, which effectively overturned all such laws in the country and made abortion on request a reality for American women, depending on the availability of services. However, many clinics set up in the wake of this historic decision have been bombed or torched by Christian vigilantes. And, in the wake of recent Supreme Court appointments and an increasingly conservative and intolerant political climate, freedom of choice on abortion in the United States may be in some jeopardy.

In 1969, Canada's old abortion statute, derived directly from England's nineteenth-century laws, was amended to allow abortions in "accredited or approved hospitals" if "continuation of the pregnancy would be or would be likely to endanger [the mother's] life or health," provided her application was approved by a therapeutic abortion committee. Few hospitals set up such committees, however, so many Canadian women were forced either to go to the United States for help or to turn to Dr. Henry Morgentaler, who, in the early 1970s, set up a clinic in Montreal. He was arrested by the then Liberal government of the province of Quebec in a fit of demographic panic when it discovered that its birth rate was the lowest in Canada. Morgentaler was acquitted at his trial, but the Quebec Court of Appeal overturned the jury verdict and ordered him to jail. This decision was appealed to the Canadian Supreme Court, where the majority decision upheld the Quebec Court of Appeal decision. Dr. Morgentaler spent ten months in jail. The section of the Criminal Code giving appeal courts such extraordinary power had never been used before in the history of Canada; the furor that arose as a response to such a gross violation of basic human rights led to that section of the code being repealed in the Canadian parliament.

But in 1989, the Canadian federal government introduced Bill C-43, which would have returned abortion to the Criminal Code of Canada, and made abortions legal only if the patient's physician was certain that continuing the pregnancy was a danger to the "health" of the woman. Gone were the hospital abortion committees; physicians were liable to spend two years in jail if they "broke" the law, presumably by performing an abortion on a woman whose health was *not* threatened by continuing the pregnancy. Since the ability to predict on a case-by-case basis how a woman would respond by being forced to remain pregnant is virtually nonexistent, the law in essence became simply a license for the anti-choice crusaders to harass physicians, which they promised to do. Bill C-43 passed the House of Commons but suffered an interesting fate in the nonelected Senate, where a tie vote brought about its defeat. Opposing the bill throughout was an uneasy "alliance" of anti- and pro-choice forces, each of whom opposed the bill for diametrically different reasons; politics does indeed make strange bedfellows.

The religious anti-choice faction in the abortion debate (the self-styled pro-lifers) is fighting the trend toward a more liberal law. Although some of the more moderate Christian denominations support the pro-choice cause, the Roman Catholic Church and the fundamentalists place great resources at the disposal of the anti-choice movement, resources without which it could not function. Large turnouts at anti-abortion rallies are always the result of pressure from the pulpit.

In spite of the church's support for the anti-choice cause, Roman Catholics continue to have abortions at a rate proportional to their representation in the total population. The church, knowing that it is losing its power to control its flock, lashes out like a dying dragon thrashing its tail, strong-arming politicians to use secular law to bolster its failing power of "friendly" persuasion.

It is foolhardy to be sanguine about the eventual outcome of the present abortion debate in the Western world. The pendulum may very easily move back to the restrictive end of the statutory continuum as it did in Romania in 1966. In 1957, a liberal law on abortion was passed in that country; as a consequence, the birth rate fell dramatically (from 22.9 per thousand population in 1957 to 14.3 in 1966). The government, in a fit of demographic panic, suddenly passed a very restrictive law making it almost impossible for a woman in Romania to interrupt a pregnancy legally. The effect on the birth rate was startling, rising to 27.3 per thousand population in 1967. Along with the increase in births—which no doubt pleased the politicians—there came an increase in both infant and maternal mortality and morbidity, due to the strain on the health care system and the increase in illegal abortions.

Anti-choice people should recognize that it would be in their best interest to work with the pro-choice groups to get the state out of the business of using the abortion law as a demographic safety valve. The state's assumption of the right to legislate this issue in the manner it does is a dangerous sword that cuts in both directions. While many good Christians work to get the federal government to pass a law prohibiting abortions, they fail to realize that the same government could, given another set of demographic conditions, pass legislation forcing women to have abortions against their will. What is now happening in China could happen here.

GENDER ROLE SOCIALIZATION

Human beings create societies which in turn foster and encourage attitudes and behaviors that proved useful in the task of forging those societies. Unfortunately, the characteristics that are appropriate to the task of creating a society may not necessarily be those that are appropriate to later stages in that society's evolution. Twentieth-century North American society is a product of nineteenth-century European expansionism, a process fueled by ruthless pronatalist policies and attitudes; such demographic aggression led to the military aggression that saw the continent populated with white Europeans before the century came to an end.

In a society committed to this kind of expansionism, certain expectations are laid on individuals, i.e., they are expected to play certain roles, many of which are linked to gender. Gender roles (also called sex roles) can be very rigidly defined with thick boundaries between those assigned to males and those assigned to females; the more rigid the boundaries, the more pressure is exerted on individuals to behave in accordance with those roles. This was the situation during the building of North America; only in the second half of the twentieth century have we begun to witness changes in gender roles for both women and men.

Larry Feldman, a researcher in family studies, has reviewed the literature on traditional gender roles and their impact on family functioning.[50] According to Feldman, women were expected in our society to be: (1) home- and child-oriented; (2) warm, affectionate, gentle, and tender; (3) aware of others' feelings, considerate, tactful, and compassionate; (4) moody, high strung, temperamental, excitable, emotional, subjective, and illogical; (5) complaining and nagging; (6) weak, helpless, fragile, and easily hurt emotionally; and (7) submissive, yielding, and dependent.

Men, on the contrary, were: (1) ambitious, competitive, enterprising, and worldly; (2) calm, stable, unemotional, realistic, and logical; (3) strong, tough, and powerful; (4) aggressive, forceful, decisive, and dominant; (5) independent and self-reliant; (6) harsh, severe, stern, and cruel; and (7) autocratic, rigid, and arrogant.

It is obvious that the characteristics assigned to women are those appropriate to the tasks of childbearing, tending the home and hearth, and supplying the emotional component of the male/female relationship; whereas those assigned to males are the ones required to fight wars, make killings in the marketplace, and return to the nest to have one's wounds licked by the nurturant partner and to impregnate her at each visit. These are the gender roles commensurate with a coercively pronatalist human society.

These traditional roles have been indicted as a major factor in marital stress. Feldman, after his review of the literature, came to the following conclusion: "Sex role conditioning exerts a variety of dysfunctional influences on the marital and family relationship; and these male and female sex roles interact in a mutually reinforcing way that inhibits the psychological development of each family member"[51]

We need to explore here how gender role socialization contributes to couple problems. As we saw in chapter 3, self-esteem derives from two sources: the type and amount of affectionate caring a child receives in early life and the manner in which caring adults facilitate the child's attempts at mastery. We pointed out that this latter activity is one that is actively discouraged by Christian doctrine; we are taught to place our reliance on God, not on our own competence and that of other human beings. If a child's sense of mastery is facilitated, he or she will grow up constantly evaluating the gender roles assigned to men and women, conforming to them where they are relevant at that point of self-development, but rejecting those aspects that run counter to a developing sense of competence and self-esteem. When social and religious influences actively interfere with this process, ego growth is stunted and the child inevitably falls back on prescribed gender roles.

When it comes time to try to form a heterosexual relationship, individuals whose sense of competence has been thwarted by familial and religious influences and who fall back on prescribed gender roles, are almost certain to fail. The man, conforming to a traditional gender role, thereby cut off from much of his potential as a human being, will have difficulty relating to his partner as a sensate being. His tendency to relate to her in terms of those characteristics assigned to women by traditional gender roles is certain to contribute to relationship problems.

A particular type of couple problem exists when the woman continues to grow psychologically after the marriage, in ways that challenge her assigned gender role. If her partner is locked into a traditional male role, showing no evidence of an inclination to challenge it, he will react negatively to his wife's attempts to self-actualize. If she wishes to finish her university degree, for example, he may construe this to mean that she is not happy with him as a husband, nor her role as a mother.

It might seem, at first glance, a little unfair to blame the Christian church for the rigid destructive gender roles from which women and men are struggling to free themselves. After all, don't we now have female priests in the Protestant churches and aren't some Roman Catholic women petitioning the Vatican for the same rights?

The fact is that, on two levels, we can justifiably lay blame at the door of the Christian church for this state of affairs. Centuries of indoctrination regarding sexuality and reproduction helped to mold these gender roles. In the fifteenth century, the *Malleus Maleficarum* expressed prevailing Christian notions about males and females, and because of its longstanding influence, helped to engrain these attitudes deeply into Western consciousness. It was noted before that women were more likely to become agents of the devil, "more ready to receive the influence of a disembodied spirit," because they were "more credulous," "more impressionable," had "slippery tongues," were "intellectually like children," "more carnal" than men, and had "weak memories." It was all quite simple: "Since [women] are feebler both in mind and body, it is not surprising that they should come more under the spell of witchcraft."[52]

Men, on the other hand, were completely free of these defects: "And blessed be the Highest Who have so far preserved the male sex from so great a crime: for since He was willing to be born and to suffer for us, therefore He has granted to men this privilege."[53]

As the agents of God, men were charged with the task of impregnating their wives as often as humanly possible. Women, even though they were judged to be "weaker in mind and body," were nonetheless expected to withstand repeated pregnancies, their punishment for being normal sexual human beings.

Not only was the Christian church responsible for laying the groundwork for explosive European population growth, but in each country the church supported the governments in their policies of demographic aggression against their own people. The Church of England stood foursquare with the British regimes during the era of Victorian expansionism, England's anti-abortion laws, and the battle against birth control. Victorian pronatalist attitudes about sexuality received strong support from churchmen. In North America, God was often used to justify the most heinous crimes against the "heathen" North American Indian. Pope Pius IX did his part in 1869 when he tightened up on the church's heretofore relaxed attitudes about abortion. In Nazi Germany, the same Roman Catholic Church allied itself with Hitler to the bitter end, in spite of his often harsh treatment of many of his fellow Catholics. Thus, there is a compelling link between the gender roles identified by workers in the field, reviewed by Feldman, and the teachings of the Christian church on sexuality and reproduction.

There are, however, signs of change. Through the feminist movement, women are becoming increasingly sensitized to the constricting impact of these traditional gender roles which have made it difficult or impossible for them to realize their full potential as human beings. Men, on the other hand, appear to be less aware of the degree to which their socialization has contributed to difficulty in establishing relationships with females, as well as to their greater tendency to develop psychosomatic illnesses.

In essence, this kind of demographic "sexploitation," inherent in the pronationalist sex code, has left men and women in Western Christian society open to many other forms of exploitation, economic and interpersonal. The resultant alienation leaves them unable to take sufficient charge of that aspect of their lives in order to withstand the manipulative strategies of the advertising huckster and the porno peddler. It also leaves people in Western society open to a wide variety of sexual and relationship problems. These issues will be examined in the next chapter.

NOTES

1. Abraham Feinberg, *Sex and the Pulpit* (Toronto: Methuen, 1981), p. 46.

2. C. A. Tripp, *The Homosexual Matrix* (New York: New American Library, 1976), p. 7.

3. W. W. Watters, J. A. Lamont, J. Askwith, and May Cohen, "Education for Sexuality: The Physician's Role," *Canadian Family Physician* 27 (December 1981).

4. Ellen Peck and Judith Senderowitz, *Pronatalism: The Myth of Mom and Apple Pie* (New York: Thomas Y. Crowell Company, 1974), p. 1.

5. Judith Blake, "Coercive Pronatalism and American Population Policy," *Preliminary Papers: Results of Current Research in Demography,* No 2. (University of California, Berkeley: International Population and Urban Research, December 1972).

6. Solomon Ganzfried, *Code of Jewish Law,* trans. Hyman E. Goldin (New York: Hebrew Publishing Company, 1927), vol. 4, chap. 150, pp. 13, 14.

7. Ibid., chap. 45, p. 6.

8. Ibid., chap. 46, p. 10.

9. Ibid., chap. 150, p. 16.

10. Ibid., chap. 151, p. 18.

11. John T. Noonan, Jr., *Contraception: The History of Its Treatment by the Catholic Theologians* (Cambridge, Mass.: The Belknap Press, 1966), p. 81.

12. Reay Tannahill, *Sex in History* (New York: Stein and Day, 1980), p. 138.

13. Ibid. p. 147.

14. Vern L. Bullough, "Introduction: The Christian Inheritance," in Vern L. Bullough and James Brundage, eds., *Sexual Practices in the Medieval Church* (Buffalo, N.Y.: Prometheus Books, 1982), p. 7.

15. Noonan, *Contraception,* p. 46.

16. *Globe and Mail* (Toronto), September 6, 1984.

17. A. Hitler, *Mein Kampf,* trans. Ralph Manheim (Boston: Houghton-Mifflin Co., 1943), p. 133.

18. Ronald and Juliette Goldman, *Children's Sexual Thinking* (London: Routledge and Kegan Paul, 1982).

19. William A. Fisher, Donn Byrne, Leonard A. White, and Kathryn Kelley, "Erotophobia–Erotophilia as a Dimension of Personality," *Journal of Sex Research* 25, no 1. (February 1988): 123–51.

20. Ernest Jones, *The Life and Work of Sigmund Freud* (New York: Basic Books), 2: 12.

21. Stevi Jackson, *Childhood and Sexuality* (Oxford: Basil Blackwell, 1982), p. 180.

22. Shere Hite, *The Hite Report on Male Sexuality* (New York: Alfred A. Knopf, 1981), p. 23.

23. James W. Prescott, "Body Pleasure and the Origins of Violence," *Bulletin of the Atomic Scientists,* November 1975, pp. 10–20.

24. Ibid., p. 13.

25. Henrich Kramer and James Sprenger, *The Malleus Maleficarum,* trans. Montague Summers (London: John Rodker, 1928; reprint New York: Dover Publications, 1971).

26. Ibid., p. 47.

27. Erwin J. Haeberle, *The Sex Atlas* (New York: Continum Press, 1982), p. 388.

28. Tannahill, *Sex in History,* p. 161.

29. Haeberle, *The Sex Atlas,* p. 199.

30. Ibid., p. 201.

31. Michael Carrera, *Sex, the Facts, the Acts, the Feelings* (New York: Crown Publishers, Inc., 1981), p. 395.

32. Goldman and Goldman, *Children's Sexual Thinking,* p. 342.

33. Haeberle, *The Sex Atlas,* p. 230.

34. Gilbert H. Herdt, *Guardians of the Flute: Idioms of Masculinity* (New York: McGraw-Hill, 1981).

35. Noonan, *Contraception,* p. 54.

36. John Boswell, *Christianity, Social Tolerance, and Homosexuality: Gay People in Western Europe from the Beginning of the Christian Era to the Fourteenth Century* (Chicago: University of Chicago Press, 1980).

37. John A. Watt, *The Zenith of the Medieval Papacy,* in Christopher Hollis, ed., *The Papacy* (New York: Macmillan, 1964).

38. Wendell W. Watters, *Compulsory Parenthood: The Truth about Abortion* (Toronto: McClelland and Stewart, 1976).

39. Boswell, *Christianity, Social Tolerance, and Homosexuality,* p. 218.

40. Noonan, *Contraception,* p. 52.

41. Philo, *De Abrahamo,* trans. F. H. Colson (Cambridge, Mass: Harvard University Press).

42. Augustine, *The Good of Marriage* 16.18, *CSEL* 41:210–11.

43. Caesarius, Bishop of Arles, Letter, in *Sermons* 1.12, *CC* 103:9.

44. Kramer and Sprenger, *Malleus Maleficarum,* p. 56.

45. Norman E. Hines, *Medical History of Contraception* (New York: Schocken Books, 1970).

46. Watters, *Compulsory Parenthood.*

47. David Yallop, *In God's Name: An Investigation into the Murder of Pope John Paul I* (London: Johnathn Cape Ltd., 1984), adduces evidence that John Paul I was murdered by archconservatives within the Vatican, who feared that the pontiff would overturn *Humanae Vitae.*

48. Bertrand Russell, *Why I Am Not a Christian* (London: Allen and Unwin, 1967).

49. John T. Noonan, Jr., "The Catholic Church and Abortion," *The Dublin Review* 241, no. 514 (1967–68): 315.

50. Larry Feldman, "Sex Roles and Family Dynamics," in Froma Walsh, ed., *Normal Family Processes* (New York: Guilford Press, 1982), pp. 354–79.

51. Ibid., p. 375.
52. Kramer and Springer, *Malleus Maleficarum,* p. 44.
53. Ibid. p. 47.

7

Christian Pronatalism and Human Sexual Suffering

"It is ironic that in spite of the churches' age-old preoccupation—one could almost say 'obsession' with sex, most churches at the official level have failed to formulate a positive theology of sex and the body. Few aspects of their combined teaching have done more harm, twisted more lives, or heaped more unnecessary guilt on millions of people than their generally negative approach to this very basic element in human life and development."
— Tom Harpur[1]

"Marriage—in a Christian civilization at least—is often a failure. On that point there can be no manner of doubt. It can be the gate of an earthly Eden but it is, in actual fact, often a hell of torment."
— Th. Van de Veld[2]

In the previous chapter, we examined the authoritarian pronatalist sex code and the role of the Christian church in shaping attitudes toward sexuality and gender identity in the Western world. In this chapter we look at specific human problems related to sexuality and reveal the part played by the pronatalist code. Areas to be examined are sexual dysfunction, relationship problems, rape, child sexual molestation, and pornography.

There are two ways of approaching these problems. We may begin by asking why these ills occur, or we may turn the whole issue on its head and ask the opposite question: What is it that protects some people from having such problems in a society as erotophobic as ours, one that encourages people to wage such constant war with themselves?

115

SEXUAL DYSFUNCTIONS

Sexual dysfunctions are those conditions in males and females which prevent them from experiencing the sexual response cycle completely. That cycle in the male consists of arousal with erection, excitation, plateau, orgasm, and resolution. In the female, it consists of arousal with vaginal lubrication, excitation, plateau, orgasm, and resolution. The principal male dysfunctions are erectile dysfunction (primary or secondary impotence*), premature ejaculation, and retarded ejaculation. The principal female dysfunctions are primary anorgasmia (never having had an orgasm) and secondary orgasm (no longer having orgasms). More recently, both in males and females, another condition has achieved the distinction of being classified as a dysfunction, namely, the loss of sexual desire.

While this is not the place for an exhaustive discussion of sexual dysfunctions, the purposes of this study will be served if we take one male and one female dysfunction and demonstrate how the pronatalist sex code has contributed to the production of each. The male dysfunction we shall discuss is *premature ejaculation,* the female *primary anorgasmia.*

The term premature ejaculation derives from the coital fixation inherent in the Christian approach to sexuality, which in turn leads to such sexual myths as the vaginal orgasm and the simultaneous orgasm. Still deeply engrained in the Western psyche is the notion that if a woman is going to have an orgasm at all, it should come during sexual intercourse and, according to sex manuals that were published well into this century, the couple's orgasm should be simultaneous.[3,4] If they cannot "climax" together, the male partner should not ejaculate until after the female partner has had her peak experience. (Note that stress is laid on ejaculation rather than orgasm, reflecting procreative, not pleasurable, concerns.)

Notwithstanding the religious origins of these myths, they were given added legitimacy when Freud incorporated them into psychoanalytic theory in a way that convinced many women that they were failures if they did not have "vaginal" orgasms; and many males became convinced that *they* were failures if they could not "give" their partner orgasms during intercourse. As recently as 1975, psychiatrist Judd Marmor defined premature ejaculation as "that condition in which a man, with any woman, achieves orgasm before or within seconds after vaginal intromission or in which a man, despite having a partner capable of achieving orgasm without difficulty, *is unable to delay his orgasm or ejaculation during intravaginal coitus for a sufficient length of time to satisfy her in at least half of their coital connections* (my italics)."[5] This defi-

---

*A male suffering from *primary impotence* has never been able to have an erection. One suffering from *secondary impotence* has lost his former ability to have an erection.

nition begs the questions, "Why one-half?" and "Why not one-quarter or three-quarters?"

Thus, premature ejaculation had the somewhat dubious distinction of being the only condition in all of medicine that was diagnosed in one person by a failure of another to react. The absurdity of the situation finally got through to those concerned about nomenclature; the DSM III (third edition of the *Diagnostic and Statistical Manual*) of the American Psychiatric Association now defines premature ejaculation as that occurring "before the individual wishes it, because of recurrent and persistent absence of reasonable voluntary control of ejaculation and orgasm during sexual activity."[6]

This deep-seated belief that the female orgasm should take place during coitus has ruined the sex lives of countless couples. Let us illustrate with a clinical example.

Case Study

A university professor and his wife, both in their mid-fifties, were referred for help with a sexual problem. From the start of their marriage, the couple's sexual life had been a source of considerable difficulty. Before marrying, they had enjoyed a wide range of noncoital sexual pleasures together, since premarital coitus was unacceptable in their American Midwest Christian community; they enjoyed oral sex and mutual manual stimulation to orgasm. It was only after marriage, when they were now "allowed" to have "the real thing," that the couple's problem began. Both felt that the wife should experience as much pleasure to orgasm with intercourse as she had with the noncoital behaviors. She began to feel inadequate as a female, and her husband accordingly felt inadequate as a lover because he could not bring his wife to orgasm during intercourse. Only rarely did she climax with intercourse, and at no time did they think of doing the pleasurable things that had marked their premarital sexual life; these, they had been encouraged to believe, should not be a part of a married couple's sex life. The bitterness engendered in their relationship over the years, stemming directly from their sexual socialization, was so great that it was impossible to help them to unlearn old attitudes and learn new, healthy ones.

At times, operating under the influence of these destructive attitudes, a woman will present as being annorgasmic because she does not have a climax during intercourse that lasts thirty seconds; at other times, her partner presents as the one with "premature ejaculation," because his partner does not have an orgasm after prolonged coitus. Physicians, who should know better, have referred couples for sex therapy, stating that the woman was "frigid" because she was not able to have an orgasm during intercourse; meanwhile, her sexual partner had no appreciation of the importance of sensuous cuddling and caressing, ignored manual genital stimulation altogether, and penetrated his partner as soon as he got an erection, ejaculating seconds later. On the other side of the coin, many men, ignorant of the fact that the average male ejaculates after two to five minutes of coitus, consider themselves "premature ejaculators" because their partners are not orgastic after ten minutes of vigorous pelvic thrusting; examination usually reveals female partners who are extemely inhibited sexually and who have never masturbated to discover their own sexual response.

RELATIONSHIP PROBLEMS: THE STORY OF KEN AND BARBARA

In chapter 6, we discussed the issue of gender role socialization and the part played by Christianity in forging the roles which have been shown to be at the root of many problems between couples. The following case history illustrates how such gender role socialization interacts with socialization around sexual issues to produce such relationship difficulties.

Ken and Barbara, a middle-class, physically attractive couple in their early thirties, had two children aged three and five. They presented with the complaint that Barbara had had, for the past three years, no interest in sex except in the few days following her period. Barbara also suffered from bouts of irritability with both Ken and the children, as well as suspicion regarding Ken's faithfulness. Following an initial diagnosis of premenstrual tension, she began receiving progesterone, but this did not relieve her symptoms. At first Ken tried to be solicitous, giving Barbara reassurance and urging her to take her medication whenever she got upset. Recently, it had become difficult for Ken to tolerate Barbara's emotional outbursts. He would often remove himself from the situation, which only made her feel more frustrated.

Since Barbara had been refusing Ken's sexual advances, he had stopped initiating sex at all but waited until she felt like it. In the initial session, he denied feeling any resentment toward Barbara since he understood that, being a woman, especially one with a "medical" problem, she couldn't really help it. Ken's resentment was directed instead at the medical profession, which had not been able to relieve Barbara's symptoms so that she would recover her interest in sex. He had been masturbating to relieve his sexual tension.

Barbara had been born into a fundamentalist religious family with very strict ideas about good behavior. As a little girl she was not allowed to have fun since that might mean getting dirty; work always came before play and being good was very important. Barbara's family had severe problems in dealing with feelings; whenever people got angry at each other, they would yell and scream but not in a way that allowed for resolution of differences. She did not like this behavior in her parents, however, and one of the reasons for

Barbara's attraction to Ken was the fact that in his family nobody ever screamed at anybody else; they were more "civilized." Barbara initially found Ken's emotionless approach to life very soothing; she often claimed he was her "rock," at least in the beginning.

Barbara's parents separated when she was in her early teens, an event that contributed a great deal to her insecurity and made her look for a man who was calm and unemotional, in sharp contrast to her father. After her parents split up, Barara's mother became very dependent on her; in fact, she and her mother developed a mutual vacillating dependency in which each played, alternately, the mother and the child. This has continued until the present time, much to the irritation of Ken, who doesn't feel that his wife should be so dependent on her mother.

Ken had been raised in a fundamentalist Christian family as well, where his father was described by him as dependable and responsible, but emotionally remote as a way of maintaining his position as head of the family. Nonetheless, Ken's father never had any doubt about what was right and wrong. Ken's mother was slightly more emotional than his father. Ken could never really talk to his father but was able to talk slightly more to his mother. He feels, however, that he was "very fortunate" to have been raised in such a "close" family, and is certain that his wife was attracted to him because of that.

Initially in the conjoint session the couple presented as having a wonderful relationship, except for Barbara's problem, which Ken saw as "medical." Barbara vacillated a great deal in terms of her own perceptions of the problem. At times, when she appeared to be under Ken's control, Barbara would agree that she was too "emotional" and should try harder to adopt her husband's stoical approach to life. At other times Barbara would assert herself and describe her real feelings about their marriage: the fact that Kenneth behaved like a robot in their interaction, would not listen to her when she got upset, and was intimate only when he wanted sexual intercourse.

At the beginning of their contact in the clinic, Ken and Barbara stated that the sexual relationship was great during those days when she wanted to have sex. However, this turned out not to be the real story. In the early part of their marriage, Barbara did not enjoy sex at all, and only gradually became orgasmic on manual stimulation.

Premarital sexual interaction rarely involved intercourse or direct manual stimulation of the genitals. Because of their Christian backgrounds, Ken and Barbara felt such direct expression of sexuality was sinful, so Ken would lie on top of Barbara, fully clothed, and simulate the movements of intercourse until the resulting friction led to orgasm. This was satisfying to her because it meant that their bodies were constantly in contact with each other, and because it took a long time for Ken to achieve orgasm. This prolonged stimulation of the clitoris usually led to orgasm.

When these noncoital sexual behaviors diminished after marriage, Barbara became less and less satisfied. Being a good Christian girl, however, she had never masturbated and had, therefore, no way of knowing what she might ask Ken to do to give her pleasure. She would never think it proper to tell him, in any case.

The circumstances surrounding the conception and birth of their two children were quite illuminating. Barbara decided she wanted to have children early in the marriage; Ken was opposed to this, preferring to wait until they had financial stability. However, they were unable to resolve their differences in any adult way. Ken simply gave in "to please her." Now when Barbara gets upset about her role as a mother, Ken throws it up to her that it was she, not he, who wanted to get right into the parenthood business.

Formulation of the Problem

Ken and Barbara had been exposed to Christian doctrine all their lives. They obviously did not have a deep interest in religion, as something to be concerned and curious about, but rather continued their association purely out of habit. In essence, they were prepared to live unexamined lives.

Ken's self-esteem was tied up with his conformity to the stereotypical male role he had seen enacted by his cold, aloof, authoritarian father. His ability to cope with ambivalence was limited; in spite of the fact that he could not talk to his father, Ken denied having any negative feelings toward him. Indeed, Ken frequently talked about how lucky he was to have been brought up in a home with no fighting. He also went to great lengths to deny his anger toward his wife, dealing with it rather by emotional withdrawal and codifying Barbara's emotional outbursts as "sick" behavior. Denial of anger and an infantile method of dealing with ambivalence are integral components of Christian teaching, as we have discussed in chapter 4.

Barbara, on the other hand, was slightly more tolerant of her negative feelings. At times she would give voice to her anger toward Ken in a very articulate way, but her self-esteem was so low that she tended to vacillate. When Ken used any of his controlling tactics on Barbara, she would regress in front of our eyes, turn the negative feelings against herself, and join Ken in codifying her emotional outbursts as "sick." Barbara's experience with her parents did not help since they appeared to be people who openly expressed anger, but not in a manner that allowed for any real adult-to-adult negotiation to take place.

Between her parents' bitter, infantile bickering and her in-laws' inability to express any anger—an option that once attracted her—Barbara seemed to be struggling to find a more adult way of coping with such negative emergency emotions in herself toward her husband. She relied excessively on Ken for her self-esteem, having received very little encouragement throughout her life to realize her own potential and to feel good about herself, independent of what anyone else said about her.

When they presented at the clinic, Barbara was the "sick" one in the relationship; otherwise, according to them both, she would be behaving in the manner Kenneth considered appropriate. Ken insisted that he was happy and was most reluctant to look at his own behavior and attitudes in a critical way. Yet there was evidence that Ken lived a pleasureless, guilt-ridden existence. He worked hard, had no close friends and no hobbies. He not only rejected all emergency feelings in himself (just as he labeled them as "sick" in his wife), but he also did not express welfare emotions when he experienced them, which was rather rare. Ken was able to open up and share a little of what was going on inside him when he and Barbara had sexual intercourse; however, his behavior afterward, when he would often not speak to Barbara for days, suggests that such pleasure had to be followed by a period of self-denial and punishment, which took the form of a sullen angry withdrawal from the source of pleasure, his wife (see chapter 5).

Ken and Barbara's sexual socialization is a typical product of our Christian society. They had no formal sex education and grew up with most of the myths generated by the pronatalist sex code. Prior to marriage, they were at first so limited in their knowledge of what they might do to give and get sexual pleasure that they initially relied on simulated intercourse, fully clothed, to orgasm. Later, however, they were able to enjoy direct manual genital stimulation. Ken and Barbara were deeply influenced by the myth of simultaneous orgasm: he would stimulate her genitals until she was "ready" and then enter her with the idea of their coming together. Barbara often complained that Ken "came too fast" after penetration, i.e., before she had had her orgasm. Only after a long time did they negotiate that he could stimulate her genitals manually to orgasm after he had his climax with intercourse.

Both were literally victims of traditional gender role socialization. Kenneth had the macho role down to a T: assertive, competitive, emotionless, and controlling. Behind the arrogant male role, however, he was lonely and frightened, constantly at war with the sensate, feeling, truly human self that had never been allowed to emerge and develop its rightful place within Ken's personality. Furthermore, he showed no signs of wanting this part of himself to emerge from behind the rigid role he played.

Barbara was brought up to be the passive, dependent, emotional little girl-woman whose fate was to spend her life being dependent on a man. She tried—at times desperately—to stay within the confines of that role. However, at times in interviews with Ken but more so when she was seen alone, the pressure to actualize her own self from behind that role was evident. When Barbara became open, she was articulate and insightful about the problems in their relationship, especially about her husband's robot-like behavior, and the legitimacy of her emotional reaction to that behavior. However, she was sensitive enough to realize that this was threatening to Ken, with his limited repertoire of human responses; hence, when he would withdraw further emotionally, Barbara would respond to this manipulation by regressing to the role of the weak, inadequate, emotionally "sick" female. She was afraid that Ken would be so threatened that he would withdraw completely from the relationship.

RAPE

It is now fashionable to view rape as primarily an act of violence perpetrated against women. It may, however, be a mistake to ignore the fact that, violent though it most certainly is, rape is also a sexual act. We should not minimize the contribution made by the sexual socialization of males and females in the act of rape.

The connection between Christian sexual indoctrination and the production of a rape mentality in men is suggested by the following example.

Case Study

A young man was in prison for rape, and gave the following story in an interview conducted to see if there was any basis for psycyhiatric treatment after his release from prison. On the fateful night, he was returning home to his wife after an evening out with the boys at a bar. But he stopped first at a house he chose at random, broke in, and raped a woman in her kitchen. When we asked if he had been sexually excited at that time, he admitted that he had been. When we asked why he hadn't simply masturbated to relieve his sexual tension, he looked horrified and replied, "Oh, I was born a Catholic . . . that's a mortal sin."

This man was not psychotic and was of average, if not above-average, intelligence. It is rather frightening to realize that he was expressing what he had obviously been socialized to believe, namely, that having sexual intercourse with a woman who did not want it was less a sin in the eyes of God than relieving his sexual tension by manually stimulating his penis.

Being a true product of Christian society, he was deeply influenced by teachings about the conflict between the "flesh" and "spirit." He had not been exposed to any sex education that would have enabled him to develop an integrated, guilt-free, enlightened attitude toward his sexuality; hence the probability that he might express his sexual needs in a situation known in advance to be associated with risk of punishment.

Rape, while indeed a sexual act, is also one of intense hostility toward women. Given the Christian intolerance of anger as a normal human emotion, our rapist had no acceptable way of dealing with his natural anger toward his wife and his mother; he tended, rather, to follow the Catholic trend of placing them all on pedestals to be worshiped in a manner similar to the virgin Mary.

Coupled with all this is the socialized tendency in males to express feelings on a behavioral level if they cannot repress them entirely. This applies to both positive and negative feelings. It is common in a couple assessment to ask each partner how they express anger to the other, only to have the man respond instantly, almost like a reflex, "I have never hit her," the behavioral level being the only one on which he can conceptualize angry feelings. The same applies to welfare emotions. Men commonly see sexual intercourse as a way of "making up" after an unresolved disagreement with their partner, and are often confused when the partner is unresponsive. Women as a rule prefer to resolve issues verbally before they can get into a mood for lovemaking.

The traditional Christian view holds that men have a God-given "right" to sexual favors from women, who are regarded as little more than the property of the man to whom they are married. Until very recently, "marital rape" was considered unthinkable; if a man has this kind of "right" with a wife, it is easy to understand why many men still assume that this right extends to other women. When we look at female sexual socialization, we find another factor that contributes to rape: this is what we might term the "Malleus Maleficarum Factor." Church teachings traditionally frowned on women acknowledging their sexual desires. Women who did admit to being interested in sex for its own sake (rather than remain mere objects by which men could satisfy their physical lust, and the church its demographic lust), would be in danger of being branded a witch and burned at the stake at worst, or at best labeled a loose woman and rejected from polite society. It is small wonder that women were forced to deal with their normal sexuality in such a deceptive manner, by pretending not to be sexual, all the while sending covert message to the right male that he should try to break through the demure putoffs that she was forced to make to his first approaches. Freud was moved to comment: "[The erotic life] of women—partly owing to the stunting effect of civilized conditions and partly owing to their conventional secretiveness and insincerity—is still veiled in an inpenetrable obscurity."[7] One of the cartoons in my collection shows a couple on a couch looking somewhat disheveled, with the woman saying to the man, "Don't give up so soon, my mother always told me to say no only twice." This patently dishonest role that women are still encouraged to play contributes to rape behavior in the male.

One investigator, after reviewing the research on social factors in rapists' behavior, stated: "It seems safe to conclude that there is nothing inherent in the socialization processes specific to Catholicism or Protestantism that precludes subsequent acts of rape."[8] Herein lies the strong suggestion that such Christian socialization actually contributes to acts of rape.

CHILD SEXUAL MOLESTATION

The issue of the sexual molestation of children is only slowly coming out from under the dense cloud of secrecy and hypocrisy. Repeated surveys have shown that 20 to 25 percent of adult females in the United States report having been sexually molested by an adult male before the age of thirteen,[9] and there is no reason to suppose that Canadian figures are any different. Nonetheless, many priests, ministers, and rabbis interviewed by one researcher all insisted that "that" did not happen in their congregation.[10]

The problem of child sexual molestation has been confounded by the issue of consanguinity, or relatedness by blood. Psychoanalysis has tended to focus on incest and the so-called incest taboo, as if the biological tie between victimizer and victim, not the sexual misuse of children, were the most important issue here. Instead of examining our society to discover the forces giving rise to this tendency, we have focused on the taboo itself. But as Paul Pruyser put it, "the strength of a taboo is commensurate with the desire it seeks to curb."[11] In fact, we would not need an "incest" taboo unless our society already had an attitude that allows child molestation, excluding close relatives. That the taboo "works" to some extent is suggested by the research of David Finkelhor, who found that female children were more likely to be sexually molested by stepfathers than by biological fathers—small comfort to the thousands of girls molested by uncles and "friendly" neighbors.[12]

Sigmund Freud, in spite of his monumental contribution to an understanding of human behavior, has, regrettably, also contributed to the misinformation surrounding this problem. Freud was initially appalled to hear stories from his female patients of sexual molestation by fathers and other adult relatives. Unable to accept that so many of the good burghers of Vienna could victimize children in this way, Freud concluded that these stories were fantasies in which the women were expressing their deep-seated oedipal longing for the father.[13] This refusal by Freud to believe his female patients is characteristic of the problem of child sexual molestation. Many young giris, when they overcome their fear and guilt enough to try to tell their mother, find, to their utter dismay, that she does not take her daughter seriously or else blames her for the seduction. The thinking behind the *Malleus Maleficarum* dies hard.

Florence Rush looked at the historical, anthropological, and religious roots of child sexual molestation and found that those roots ran deep.[14] At the base of the problem was the belief in both the Jewish and Christian tradition that wives and daughters were the property of the men who owned them; the rape of a virgin, therefore, was not a crime against the woman (or girl) herself but against her owner. The man's property was thereby "spoiled" unless the seducer agreed to marry her. In this case, the female's marketability counted most in determing the scope of the crime of child rape.

During the witch hunts that followed the publication of the *Malleus Maleficarum,* thousands of children throughout Europe were burned at the stake as witches for having copulated with the devil. In France, a 6-year-old was considered old enough to give consent to intercourse. In what must be the most heinous example of blaming the victim, children were often molested by adult males and subsequently burned at the stake as witches; it was commonly held that since men could not be witches, they must have been victims of diabolical sexual seduction by the female children. Although we no longer burn these children at the stake, we still often blame them for their own victimization.

Complementing these social factors that place blame on the victims of sexual abuse are the ways men are socialized around sexuality itself and their gender role. Sandra Butler, speaking about incest specifically, put it in this way: "We study them, we analyze them, and we punish them, and still we fail to understand that male incestuous aggressors are, in all too many ways, the products of our society's belief about maleness."[15] In the vast majority of cases, the child molester is a male; women rarely molest children sexually. The victims are predominantly female (19.2 percent in Finkelhor's study), although males do not escape (8.6 percent).

Many attempts have been made to uncover what characterizes men who molest children, most of the work having been done in connection with incest cases. A number of factors have been cited: mental retardation, psychosis, alcoholism, and psychopathy have all been found in men who molest children. Yet the majority of pedophiles do not suffer from these conditions. However, a history of emotional and economic deprivation is often found. A great many victimizers report a poor relationship with their own fathers, who were often absent physically or emotionally, or else brutal and authoritarian in their behavior with their children. Many victimizers were themselves brutalized as children, sexually as well as physically and psychologically. Some come from backgrounds where incest was almost the norm. Many men have poor job histories, but an equal number are regarded as stable members of the community. Most victimizers have poor social relationships outside the home.

Insufficient attention has been paid in the research literature to two very important factors; namely, the nature of the sexual relationship between the male victimizer and his adult female partner, and the issue of sexual and gender role socialization.[16] Where researchers have addressed these issues, they have found very poor sexual relationships between the man and his female partner as well as evidence of stereotypical gender role socialization. These men tend to have a very fixed traditional attitude concerning how males should behave, especially toward women, attitudes often shared by the wife as well. In fact, many of them appear straight out of the Bible with their proprietary notions about their womenfolk. Many researchers report that the victimizer often comes from a very religious family, with marked preoccupation with God, sin, and punishment. They usually give the impression on one level of being very macho and powerful, but on another very much controlled by their passive, compliant, whining wives. Some studies report these men to be "hypersexual," intensely preoccupied with sex and requiring frequent orgasms: characteristics often found in sexually insecure males.

Case Study

One couple interviewed in depth insisted that their sexual relationship was fine, although the husband had been convicted of sexually molesting two of his stepdaughters. In reply to the couple's insistence on the good state of their sexual relationship, I said that I found this hard to believe since the husband had had to go elsewhere for his sexual satisfaction. "Yes," the wife answered, "that's what makes it so strange; I never refused him." On closer questioning, however, she stated she had never been orgasmic, and often did not want to engage in sexual intercourse; but since her religious mother had told her that she should never say no to her husband, she had always gone along. For his part, he was finally able to admit that his wife's passivity during lovemaking had been a problem for him. They had never talked together about any aspect of their sexual relationship.

The following scenario illustrates one configuration of factors in a family in which the father sexually molests his own daughter. The husband—whom we call Adam—came from a family with a remote, authoritarian, Bible-thumping, punitive father, and a mother who doted on her son to meet her own unmet needs for affection from a male. Adam grew up totally unable to reconcile the demands of the role society expected him to play and the one he played in his family; Adam's mother was excessively affectionate, to the point of infantilizing him even further than did the church he was forced to attend every Sunday. Adam grew up expecting that affection from a woman was his literally by a kind of divine right, for which he had to give nothing in return. In other words, between the Christian church and his mother, Adam grew up a caricature of a man on the outside and a whining infant below the surface. His wife—let's call her Eve—on the other hand, grew up longing for a father to love her; Eve had for a maternal role model a mother who did her Christian duty by submitting sexually to her husband and having by him many babies whom she dutifully raised in the church.

Adam and Eve got married. Adam, expecting his wife to be not only a loving, doting, mothering type but also an exciting sexual partner, quickly became disillusioned on both counts. Each came to the other with totally unrealistic expectations: he expecting her to take up where his mother left off, and she expecting from him the affection she never got from her father.

Their sexual socialization added to the problems. Adam's "sex education" was full of destructive myths, including the double sex standard, coital orgasms, and the myth that men did not need sensuous pleasures. Being a good Christian girl, Eve had never masturbated and knew very little about her body. Although she was anorgasmic, she did not feel that this was a problem since her mother had told her that sex with her husband was one of the burdens of being a Christian wife. However, her lack of sexual responsiveness and the whining way in which she communicated to her husband that he was not meeting many of her needs, gradually made Adam withdraw sullenly from her. Not having the social skills to go outside the family for sex or affection, and feeling that since he got so much affection from his own family (i.e., his mother) when he was growing up, Adam was convinced that he should get it from within his own family now. When Adam's stepdaughter began to show him the normal affection a little girl feels for her father, he looked to her more and more for the affection his mother had showered on him and which his wife now denied him. Soon the need for affection became merged with his sexual needs; as a result, the child became yet another victim of the pattern of sexual and gender role socialization fostered by Christian doctrine.

PORNOGRAPHY

No two people seem to agree on a definition of pornography and whether a particular work of literature or film is pornographic. One dictionary defines pornography as "obscene literature, art or photography, especially that having little or no artistic merit."[17]

Views of what is pornographic depend on the reaction in the minds of readers or viewers. An individual who is deeply conflicted about sexuality will respond in one way to erotica; another who is reasonably comfortable with his or her sexuality will respond in an entirely different manner. Stimulated by a literary passage or a scene in a film, the sexually conflicted individual will perceive this arousal as a threat and react (or overreact) negatively to it. Obscenity vigilantes, self- as well as government-appointed, fall into this category.

The novel *Catcher in the Rye*[18] is, for most people, a delightfully sensitive book about adolescence; for others it is obscene and offensive. For many people, the German film *The Tin Drum* was a wonderful adaptation of the Gunter Grass novel[19]; the Ontario Film Censor Board, however, thought that it was too dirty to be shown in that province's movie theaters. Parenthetically, if such films as this are so harmful, how do film censors view all that obscene material without, apparently, becoming sex maniacs or going insane? If this doesn't affect them, why are they then so sure it would be harmful to other adults in the community?

It is important to make a distinction between erotica and pornography. Erotica may be collectively defined as those materials that individuals and couples use to enhance the enjoyment of their sexuality; we can cite a parallel with eating, where the ambiance, the music, and the pre-dinner cocktail are used to increase the pleasure of a good meal. Pornography, on the other hand, consists of erotic materials that contain an element of exploitation, violence, and degradation, usually of women; the term pornography should be reserved for the depiction of sexual acts that incorporate such dehumanizing features. To use another culinary metaphor, erotica may be thought of as a dinner in a fine restaurant while pornography is a junk-food meal at a fast food joint.

In Canada, the distinction between pornography and erotica has been completely lost on federal politicians who have introduced legislation into the House of Commons that defines pornography as "any visual matter showing vaginal, anal or oral intercourse, ejaculation, sexually violent behavior, bestiality, incest, necrophilia, masturbation or other sexual activity."[20] Only severely erotophobic legislators could couple masturbation and vaginal intercourse with sexually violent behavior and bestiality; and even though signs are that the legislation may not pass, the embarrassing fact of its existence demonstrates the distorted, bizarre attitudes of many politicians when it comes to sexuality.

Many find pornography exploitative and distasteful. No evidence exists, however, that even hard-core pornography has a directly harmful effect on society.[21] Unpleasant though it may be to contemplate, there is even some evidence that exposure to erotica and pornography may have a "safety-valve" effect. One controlled study has demonstrated that institutionalized rapists and child sexual molestors have less than average exposure to erotic materials during their formative years.[22]

The U.S. Commission on Obscenity and Pornography, established by President Richard Nixon in 1970, could find nothing to suggest that exposure to erotic or pornographic materials had any deleterious impact on individuals or on societies. Of the eighteen commissioners, twelve voted for the majority recommendation that "federal, state, and local legislation prohibiting the sale, exhibition, and distribution of sexual materials to consenting adults should be repealed." Of the six commissioners who voted against the recommendation, three were clergymen, one was Attorney General of California, one a lawyer who headed an organization known as Citizens for Decent Literature, and the last a woman who was generally favorable to the majority recommendation but nervous about total repeal. President Nixon duly rejected the recommendation. Two years of hard work and two million dollars went down the drain when, for obvious political purposes, the president reinforced the prevailing erotophobic attitudes of the Christian establishment.[23] In doing this, the president ignored the evidence from Denmark where erotic material of all kinds, including hard-core pornography, went on sale to the public in 1965. A significant reduction in sex crimes, especially in child sexual molestation, followed.[24]

The battle to suppress pornography legally is being fought mainly by two groups, the Christian vigilantes and some radical feminists who feel that exploitative pornography encourages men to continue to degrade women. Both groups have entirely different motives for wanting to suppress pornography. The Christian vigilantes wish to include all forms of erotica, whether or not it is pornographic, just as they oppose sex education in the schools. Among the feminists are many who favor sex education and are certainly not opposed to healthy erotica, but who object to the depiction of women as brutalized sex objects.

Hard-core pornography constitutes a powerful mirror for us to see the ugliness that exists in the ways men and women in our Christian society are socialized to relate to each other. Unfortunately, breaking the mirror will not make the ugliness go away; rather, it will only make it more difficult for the real causes of that ugliness to be identified and eradicated. It is difficult for some feminists to see that by promoting a kind of feminist Comstock Law, they are playing into the hands of those very forces in our society that have created the situation. We should ask, rather, why a market for pornography exists in the first place. For many males, especially young ones, the attraction to pornography is to learn. Much of the popularity of so-called skin magazines is that they provide the education denied to young people by Christian-dominated educational systems.

Hard-core pornography, in essence, provides men with an opportunity to "enjoy" sex in the dehumanized way our society fosters. Encouraged to deny their capacity for sensuousness, to express their emotions behaviorally rather than verbally with people close to them, to be cool but aggressive, competitive with men and dominant with women, men find themselves completely at war with their essential humanity. Being unable to harmonize their true human natures with the demands of the male role forced on them by society, they give up trying to effect a satisfying sexual relationship with a real live woman and settle instead for dehumanized, ersatz sex. The underlying Christian view of the essential sinfulness of sex is added to the diminished self-esteem stemming from men's inability to enjoy an intimate relationship with a woman. The expectation laid on them to be responsible for arousing women's dormant sexuality adds to the yoke of maleness and weighs men down even further. Since they are, in their own eyes, morally bad and inadequate to boot, it is only appropriate for them to seek release in a setting that coincides with this debased evaluation of themselves. Men wish to degrade women because deep inside they feel divided and inadequate.

While women may be the main victims of the exploitation in hard-core pornography, it is a mistake to ignore the fact that men are also exploited. In a Canadian film about pornography titled *Not a Love Story* (which, incidentally, the Ontario Board of Censors also refused to allow into commercial theaters), there is a scene in which a woman masturbates before a window with two-way communication. A sliding panel covering the window moves up when the male patron on the other side of the window puts his money in a slot. While the woman simulates masturbation, she engages in sexually provocative conversation with the man as he masturbates. As the interaction progresses, the panel keeps coming down, forcing the patron to keep the money flowing. At a certain point in the film, the camera moves to catch the faces of the men behind the glass; their expressions are the antithesis of pleasure, a powerful study in emptiness and loneliness.

Who is exploiting whom here? One could say that the "male-dominated system" is exploiting the woman by forcing her to do this sort of work. One could also say that the woman is exploiting the man by being so calculatingly provocative, or, with little fear of contradiction, that the porno merchants are exploiting them both. But the real villain, given our argument in this chapter, is the Christian church. By exploiting the human sexual drive for centuries in order to maximize its reproductive potential, by promoting a sex code that alienates people from their sexuality through guilt induction, by opposing sex education, by fostering a pattern of gender role socialization that makes it difficult for males and females to relate to each other, Christianity has created a climate that is quite favorable to exploitation by the porno merchants.

CONCLUSION

The phobic attitudes described in this chapter, which stem directly from the operation of the auhoritarian pronatalist sex code, have been deeply engrained in Western society by the teachings of the Christian church over the past sixteen centuries. Given this inescapable fact, it is likely that real changes will only take place when this code has been replaced by a healthier one (to be discussed in chapter 12).

Thus far we have discussed many aspects of Christian doctrine and shown how that doctrine conflicts with many of the principles of sound health and satisfying human relationships. In the next chapter we shall examine the possible role that Christian teachings play in the genesis of the two most serious psychiatric illnesses, depression and schizophrenia.

NOTES

1. Tom Harpur, *Heaven and Hell* (Toronto: Oxford Universities Press, 1983), p. 107.

2. Th. H. Van de Veld, *Ideal Marriage: Its Physiology and Technique* (London: William Heinmann, 1953), p. 1.

3. Ibid., p. 158.

4. Alfred Henry Tyrer, *Sex, Marriage, and Birth Control* (Toronto: Marriage Welfare Bureau, 1943), p. 164.

5. Judd Marmor, "Impotence and Ejaculatory Disturbances," in Alfred M. Freedman, Harold I. Kaplan, and Benjamin J. Sadock, eds., *Comprehensive Textbook of Psychiatry* (Baltimore: The Williams and Wilkins Company, 1975), 2:1526.

6. American Psychiatric Association, *Diagnostic and Statistical Manual of Mental Disorders,* 3rd ed. (DSM-III) (1980), p. 280.

7. Sigmund Freud, *Three Essays on Sexuality,* in James Strachey, trans. and ed., *The Complete Psychological Works of Sigmund Freud* (London: Hogarth Press, 1964), 7:151.

8. Park Elliott Dietz, "Social Factors in Rapist Behavior," in Richard T. Rada, ed., *Clinical Aspects of the Rapist,* Seminars in Psychiatry, ed. Milton Greenblatt (New York: Grune and Stratton, 1978), p. 85.

9. David Finkelhor, *Sexually Victimized Children* (New York: The Free Press, 1979), p. 132.

10. Sandra Butler, *Conspiracy of Silence: The Trauma of Incest* (San Francisco: New Glide Publications, 1978), p. 8.

11. Paul W. Pruyser, "The Seamy Side of Current Religious Beliefs," *Bulletin of the Menninger Clinic* 41, no 4 (July 1977): 343.

12. Finkelhor, *Sexually Victimized Children,* p. 88.

13. Jeffrey Moussaieff Masson, *The Assault on Truth: Freud's Supression of the Seduction Theory* (New York: Farrar, Straus and Giroux, 1984).

14. Florence Rush, *The Best Kept Secret: Sexual Abuse of Children* (Engelwood Cliffs, N.J.: Prentice-Hall, Inc., 1980).

15. Butler, *Conspiracy of Silence,* p. 65.

16. Karin C. Meiselman, *Incest* (San Francisco: Jossey-Bass, Inc., 1978).

17. *The Random House Dictionary of the English Language* (1971 ed.).

18. J. D. Salinger, *Catcher in the Rye* (New York: Bantam Books, 1952).

19. Gunter Grass, *The Tin Drum,* trans. Ralph Manheim (Middlesex, England: Penguin Books, 1961).

20. Michael Barrett, "Sex Educators and Bill C-54," *SIECCAN [Sex Information and Education Council of Canada] Newsletter* 23, no 1 (Spring 1988).

21. William A. Fisher, "The Empleror Has No Clothes; on the Fraser and Badgley Committees' Rejection of Social Science Research on Pornography," in S. Gavigan, M. A. Jackson, J. Lowman, and T. S. Palys, eds., *Regulating Sex: An Anthology of Commentaries on the Findings and Recommendations of the Badgley and Fraser Reports* (Vancouver: Simon Fraser University Press, 1986), pp. 161–75.

22. M. J. Goldstein, "Exposure to Erotic Stimuli and Sexual Deviance," *Journal of Social Issues* 29 (1973): 197–219.

23. Morris A. Lipton, "Pornography," in *Comprehensive Textbook of Psychiatry*, pp. 1594–99.

24. B. Kutchinsky, "Pornography and Its Effects in Denmark and the United States: A Rejoinder and Beyond," *Comparative Social Research* 8 (1985): 301–330.

8

Christianity and Major Psychiatric Illness

"The family, however, is merely the place where the general pathology of the culture is incubated, concentrated and finally transmuted into individual psychosis . . . the family merely distills into a lethal dose what exists in the culture at large."

—Jules Henry[1]

"Christianity . . . can be seen as promoting pathology, first by teaching that it is unavoidable and then making sure that it is in fact unavoidable by commanding its adherents to be without sin, to measure themselves against a humanly unobtainable goal of perfection."

—Roger J. Sullivan[2]

A man in his late twenties was brought by his family to the emergency room of a general hospital because he had been causing trouble among his friends, haranguing them incessantly about religion. Born a Protestant but a recent convert to Catholicism, he had been calling on his friends unannounced and telephoning repeatedly, to remind them about their wickedness and need for salvation. After the patient had been seen by the on-call psychiatric resident in the hospital, a diagnosis of paranoid schizophrenia was made and he was committed to the inpatient psychiatric unit. The young man refused to talk with the staff on the unit because he was certain they were all infidels and nonbelievers. He did, however, agree to be interviewed by the attending psychiatrist if a Roman Catholic priest were present. After making many phone calls, the psychiatrist managed to persuade one elderly semi-retired cleric to help out in this way. I was also asked to sit in on the interview as an observer, and when the priest, a short nervous man arrived, we adjourned to the interview room on the ward. The nurse went to bring the patient to us.

The patient, of average build, had marred his natural good looks by a bizarre haircut. He strode briskly into the room ahead of the nurse, and not waiting for introductions moved quickly to stand in front of the seated priest, who cowed visibly. Towering over him, the patient began a catechetical questioning of the frightened cleric, pointing and shaking his finger all the while. "Do you believe in God the Father?" he asked, to which the priest responded by nodding vigorously and muttering "I do." The catechizing continued: "And do you believe in Jesus Christ, his only son, our Lord?" More vigorous noddings and mutterings from the priest, his white knuckles gripping the arms of the chair as if he were on a roller coaster. Energized, the patient went on, "And do you believe that Christ died on the cross to save us from our sins?" By this time the churchman was nodding continuously, perspiration beginning to appear on his neck above his white collar. Was this catechist a reincarnation of Torquemada, the dreaded head of the Spanish Inquisition?

At this point, the patient stopped abruptly, lowered his arm, saying "Thank you, Father," turned on his heels and left the room. Soon after, we said goodbye to a very relieved cleric.

This strange confrontation between patient and priest resonated with meaning and significance beyond immediate comprehension. Regardless of the diagnostic label one attaches to this man, how did he come to end up behaving in such a bizarre fashion? What "caused" his "illness"? Could there be a connection between the craziness of the patient and the creed he shared with the priest? Had the "victim," turning the tables, confronted his "victimizer"?

The psychiatrist with a biological orientation would be likely to postulate a genetically transmitted biochemical disorder involving neurochemical transmitters, the substances responsible for sending messages from one nerve ending to the other in various parts of the brain. For the purely biologically oriented psychiatrist, the religious preoccupations of the patient would be fortuitous, of no etiological significance, and merely surface preoccupations of a "mind" diseased by other causes.

The more psychologically minded psychiatrist, looking at the man from a psychodynamic perspective, would be inclined to view his problem more in terms of very early emotional conflict in the areas of basic trust, autonomy, and indentity formation—the result of unsatisfactory, maladaptive interaction patterns with caring adults. For psychiatrists in this latter group, the religious preoccupations of the patient might point to deep-seated unresolved ambivalence in the relationship with his father.

Other mental health care workers would want to explore the family and other social systems in which the man was embedded, for the presence of fixed patterns of communication and negotiation—patterns so maladaptive that the patient's "breakdown" could be interpreted as an almost inevitable outcome of these chronic pathological systems.

Another conceptual model that informs the approach of most psychiatrists and psychologists is that of *learning theory*. This theory postulates that people's behavior is largely the end result of a series of conditioned responses which occur when a stimulus producing a certain response is repeatedly paired with another stimulus that would normally not produce a response of that kind, but which by association comes to do so. Within learning theory, the term *operant conditioning* is applied to situations in which certain random or emergent behaviors in the developing individual are externally rewarded, thereby increasing the likelihood that such behaviors will be repeated. Analogously, animals are trained to do tricks by rewarding only those spontaneously occurring behaviors that tend toward the desired behavior.

Operant conditioning becomes particularly important in human development in the growing child when new behaviors emerge spontaneously, behaviors that, however rudimentary, point in the direction of growth and adaptation. The reaction of caring adults at this point becomes very important. If, for example, they respond with apprehension instead of approval when the child takes his first shaky step, he is less likely, at least at first, to repeat that step. If a child shows signs of having an inquiring mind by raising questions about God and religion at an early are, that mind will be more likely to grow if the child is encouraged to reflect and examine rather than merely believe.

Despite the fact that most psychiatrists and psychologists are familiar with the concepts of learning theory, and many use these concepts freely in the various behavioral treatments, little attention has been paid to the role of society's core beliefs in the production of illness. There are many reasons for this, the chief one being that the various elements of a society's belief system are embedded deeply in its institutions as well as in the unquestioned acceptance of a wide variety of social attitudes and behaviors. As someone once said, "The last thing the fish is aware of is the salt in the water in which he swims."

The behavioral scientist Albert Ellis has concluded that there exists an irrefutable causal relationship between religion and emotional and mental illness. Dr. Ellis makes a distinction, however, between religiosity, which he associates with emotional ill health, and "mild religion," which he regards as less destructive. Ellis identifies eleven characteristics of religiosity that run counter to the development of sound mental health, characteristics that mirror many of our own. Adherence to a religious view of life, in contrast to the scientific humanist view, discourages self-acceptance, self-interest, and self-directedness, which are all necessary for sound mental and emotional functioning.

Moreover, Ellis contends, religion tends to make healthy human-to-human relationships difficult, and encourages intolerance of others and inflexibility. Seriously religious people have difficulty accepting the real world and trying to change what can be changed for the better; especially problematical is the acceptance of ambiguity and uncertainty. Religious people make use of scientific thinking, but only until it comes too close to areas that threaten their religious beliefs. They are also prone to fanatical commitments, in contrast to the less fanatical but nonetheless passionate commitments of emotionally healthy nonbelievers. Generally speaking, emotionally stable people are more inclined to be risk-takers in the sense, first of all, of recognizing what they want and then taking appropriate risks to pursue their personal goals. Deeply religious individuals, by contrast, are more inclined to feel too guilty to pursue their goals, since self-sacrifice is such an important component of their world view.[3]

GENETIC AND SOCIAL FACTORS BEHIND THE DEVELOPMENT OF MAJOR PSYCHIATRIC DISORDERS

Schizophrenia and depression (or, to use more modern nomenclature, schizophrenic and depressive disorders) together constitute the source of considerable human suffering and contribute to much of the work load of the average psychiatrist, if not also the family physician.

Some investigators continue to hold the view (and the hope?) that further research will demonstrate that genetic biological factors are solely responsible for the genesis of these conditions. This view is not discouraged by the pharmaceutical industry, which supplies so much of the funding for biological research of this kind. Most authorities in the field take the position that while a genetic predisposition may be operating in both sets of disorders, certain suprabiological factors operating in the postnatal, interpersonal, sociocultural environment must interact with the genetic "predisposition" in order for the clinical illness to appear. This intimate connection between the biological and suprabiological environment is not confined to mental illness. Since not everyone who smokes cigarettes develops lung cancer, this suggests differences in biological susceptibility; for the same reason not everyone falls victim during epidemics of highly infectious diseases. Examples of the same genetic-environmental interaction come readily to mind from fields outside of health care. A child may be born with innate musical ability or athletic potential; but these latent talents must be recognized and encouraged by the environment in order for the child to become a competent musician or athlete.

When it comes to major psychiatric illnesses, we may look at this genetic-environmental interaction in two ways. The usual assumption is that certain individuals are genetically predisposed to develop depression or schizophrenia, and that certain noxious elements in the social and interpersonal environment must be present for the illness to manifest itself.

However, the genetic contribution may not consist of an innate predisposition to develop a specific form of pathology, but rather a limitation in adaptive potential. Where this inborn capacity to master each successive developmental stage of life is limited, it may require a superhuman level of parenting skills and an absence of severe life stresses to prevent the individual from becoming psychiatrically ill. At the other end of the continuum, an individual born with an abundance of this genetically determined characteristic may master each developmental stage and cope with life's stresses very well, even if the family of origin is not very facilitative. Since the relationship between parent and child is a dynamic, interactive one, a child with limited potential for adaptation, as in the case of mental retardation or some other disability, places a strain on the caretaking skills of the parent. By contrast, a child with adaptive potential to spare may make parents with modest parenting skills look good.

The vast majority of individuals fall somewhere between the two extremes in terms of their capacity to self-actualize, i.e., to master each developmental stage and cope adaptively with stress. Hence, we are all irrevocably at the mercy of the interdependence of genetic endowment and environmental influence.

It may be helpful for our purposes to modify the foregoing analysis and postulate the following: operating in the sociocultural environment are forces that tend to make it difficult for people to grow up psychologically. These pathogenic influences act on the growing child through the medium of the family. The variability of individuals in terms of their genetically determined capacity to neutralize these influences at successive developmental stages, may exist in accordance with the ubiquitous bell-shaped curve. (Note that this is not the same thing as dichotomizing the world into those who are born with a genetic predisposition to major psychiatric illness and those who are not.)

Just as individuals vary a great deal in terms of their innate adaptive potential, so do families in terms of their ability to mediate between the wider sociocultural environment and the growing child in a way that neutralizes those pathogenic social influences that tend to compromise adaptive development. Parents with exceptionally high levels of parenting skills might be able to create a family environment in which a child with minimal innate adaptive potential could develop sufficient coping skills to enable him or her to live without developing a psychiatric illness. Conversely, a child with high levels of potential for adaptation might succumb to some form of psychiatric illness if born into a family in which the parents themselves have been severely damaged by the pathogenic forces operating in society. In the vast majority of instances, good "mental" health is dependent on the interaction between the genetic givens in the area of potential for adaptation and the family's ability to act both as a catalyst in fostering this adaptive potential and as a neutralizer of the more destructive messages coming from society at large.

SCHIZOPHRENIC DISORDERS

Psychosis has been defined as "a withdrawal from an active attempt to reconcile reality with an inner world of disorganized thinking and feeling."[4] Schizophrenia is the most common form of psychosis.

The schizophrenic disorders are conditions in which the individual patient manifests severe disturbances in perception, cognition, speech, emotional life, and behavior. Disturbances of perception, cognition, and speech include hallucinations, delusions, loosenings of associations, excessive concreteness and symbolism, incoherence, neologisms (making up words), mutism, echolalia (repeating words spoken by others), verbigeration (word repetition), and stilted language. Disturbances in the area of emotion include inappropriate emotional responses, abnormal emotions, reduced emotional response, and anhedonia (the absence of pleasure in performing any function that would normally produce pleasure). Disturbances of behavior include echopraxia (mimicking the movements of others), other forms of bizarre behavior, stuporous states, automatic obedience or automatic negativism, stereotyped behaviors, deteriorated appearance and manners, and social withdrawal. Variability in the pattern of symptoms is also a feature.

In chapter 4 we discussed the gradual transition from the stage of infantile narcissism through a long period of dependency to the adult stage of related individuation. It is in the early stages of that long developmental journey that the traveler develops the perceptual and cognitive template that shapes development on the behavioral level and influences the rest of his life; the factors determining the soundness of that template are neurological development and interaction with caring adults. If the former proceeds normally and the latter is facilitative, perceptual and cognitive development should proceed without difficulty. If the interaction with parents is nonfacilitative, the risk of developing a serious psychiatric disorder increases. It may be that the more nonfacilitative this interaction is, the greater the likelihood that the child will subsequently develop schizophrenia rather than one of the depressive disorders.

ENVIRONMENTAL SCHIZOPHRENOGENICITY

Initially, the search for schizophrenogenicity (i.e., the development of schizophrenia) in the environment focused on the mother, whose characteristics were variously cited as an excess of anxiety, hostility to the child, passivity, indifference, insensitivity to the child's needs, an inability to be physically and emotionally close to the child, and overpossessiveness. She was considered solely responsible for the child's derailed development on the long road from the stage of infantile narcissism to the stage of related individuation.

With the advent of family therapy, attention has shifted from the mother to the marital relationship and to the entire family as a semiclosed system that, within sociocultural limits, develops its own rules about how people should relate to each other. Researchers in the field have been mainly interested in family patterns of communication, negotiation, and support, especially the degree to which such patterns facilitate or discourage the establishment of ego boundaries, self-esteem, and adaptive behavior. Theodore Lidz, in summarizing his own theory, is essentially talking about the entire field when he states:

> There are two interrelated aspects of the theory. The first has to do with how the parental personalities and the transactions within the family prevent a child from differentiating adequately from the mother, separating from the family, and gaining sufficiently coherent integration to achieve an ego identity, a capacity for intimacy, and the ability to become reasonably self-sufficient by the end of adolescence. The second has to do with the development of the cognitive disorder that forms the critical attribute of the category of mental disorders we designate as schizophrenic.[5]

A variety of disturbances in the communication, negotiation, and support styles have been identified. Mixed messages in which the child receives diametrically opposed directives from a parent are commonly cited. An example is where the mother says to the child, "You can go out and play if you want to," but in a martyr-like tone designed to make the child feel guilty about not staying in and helping with the chores. Then there is the "double bind," in which a child is given a directive containing a built-in negation of that directive ("I order you to disobey me"). This represents a very destructive form of communication. Lyman Wynne and his colleagues have discovered parental communication deviance to be a consistent feature of the families of schizophrenics, especially of those patients who show marked thought disorders.[6]

Lidz has identified two categories of schizophrenogenic families. In *schizmatic* families, "The two parents are in abiding conflict, undercutting the worth of the other to the child, and the child is not only used to complete a parent's life and salvage the marriage but his psychic structure is also torn apart by the internalization of two irreconcilable parents." In *skewed* families, "One parent, usually the mother, does not establish boundaries between herself and the child, uses the child to complete her life, and continues to be extremely intrusive into the child's life, though impervious to the child's needs and feelings as a separate individual, behavior not countered by a passive spouse."[7]

Wynne has coined the term "pseudomutuality" to describe the behavior of a family in which conflicts between parents, however intense, are never allowed to surface. Family members are expected to relate to each other in accordance with externally imposed roles rather than in accordance with genuine thoughts and feelings. The presumably genetically susceptible individual in such a family manifests schizophrenic symptoms when these brittle, rigid, nongenuine role relationships break down under stress.[8]

CHRISTIAN DOCTRINE AND SCHIZOPHRENOGENICITY

Earlier in this volume I attempted to show that Christian doctrine and teachings are incompatible with many of the components of sound mental health, notably self-esteem, self-actualization and mastery, good communication skills, related individuation and the establishment of supportive human networks, and the development of healthy sexuality and reproductive responsibility. The impact of traditional gender role socialization on a relationship has also been discussed. When the couple are not only partners to each other but parents to children in a family, the destructive impact of traditional gender role socialization and the dehumanizing effects of Christian doctrine combine to compromise the healthy development of yet another generation.

It is little wonder that the mother has long been blamed for the genesis of schizophrenia. Christian doctrine, in spite of the attempts of revisionists, blames Eve for humankind's ejection from the Garden of Eden. In *Malleus Maleficarum* this guilt was reinforced: women were viewed as creatures of pure carnality, and because of their innate weakness and inferiority more likely to succumb to the blandishments of the devil.

Until recently, women in our society were not encouraged to look upon themselves as autonomous individuals capable of developing their human potential in whatever direction it took them. Even their identities were submerged in that of their husbands. (When I was a boy at school, I was taught that one should never address a letter to Mrs. Mary Blank but always to Mrs. John Blank.) Nonetheless, women were somehow expected to be effective catalysts in the self-actualization of their own children. But how can a woman be expected to develop the adaptive potential of her own biological offspring if her own adaptive potential has been compromised, not only by the gender role she has been obliged to play but by many other teachings inherent in Christian doctrine. Consider the tendency of Christian indoctrination to produce self-loathing, guilt over pleasure, the inability to be in charge of one's own sexuality and reproductivity, and a built-in orientation away from human support systems and toward the divine. Could anyone design a more inefficient training program for parents? The fact that most mothers in our society do not raise schizophrenic children has more to do with the innate humanity and good judgment of most women, and their ability to defend themselves against the more destructive effects of Christian doctrine, even when they may repeat that doctrine like parrots Sunday after Sunday.

In the authoritarian pronatalist sex code to which the Christian church still subscribes in large measure, there is one female characteristic that comes to the rescue and possibly saves many a child from serious psychiatric illness: the mother is expected to be "emotional" and allowed to be demonstrably affectionate. This is a characteristic that has long been denied to men. The male role did not call for his involvement in the initial nurturing of the infant; this was clearly "women's work." While he could play with the children when they were capable of interacting with him, the father played little part in the earlier processes of training them to interact. It is little wonder, then, that so many psychiatric patients, and not just schizophrenics, report their fathers as being more remote figures than their mothers. Coupled with this is the traditional pressure on the male to control his feelings as much as possible, to express them behaviorally if he cannot control them but never to attempt to express them verbally and directly. This is true both of emergency emotions and welfare emotions. The longing for contact with a male God may be a reflection of this longing for contact with an earthly father denied to most people in the Western world because of the roles males have been and still are encouraged to play.

To illustrate how Christian doctrine can contribute indirectly to the development of schizophrenia in a child born with limited capacity to adapt, let us construct a hypothetical scenario of the first two years of a child's life with parents Jack and Jill.

Jill got pregnant when she and Jack were deciding whether or not to get married. Since they both came from good Christian backgrounds, the idea of abortion was out of the question; therefore, the pregnancy determined the matter for them. Both felt very guilty about having had sex before they were married; because of their beliefs, they had not considered contraceptive methods.

The baby was a healthy boy whom they named Jake. They loved him very much and Jill was able to suppress, though not get entirely rid of, her resentment about having been forced into a marriage. Having been raised in a home where women were clearly looked upon as being less important than men, Jill had never been able to develop a sense of self-esteem or self-worth from mastering any challenge. Although she was reasonably bright and did well academically at school, the family attitude was that this was really a frill for a female who would one day marry and have babies. Jill had been attracted to Jack because he seemed so "strong," never getting upset over things.

From the start Jill began having difficulty in her mothering role; she worried constantly about whether or not she was a good mother. Her lack of self-esteem stemming from her socialized role as a woman, her guilt about having sex before she was married and about her resentment at being forced to get married, not to mention the guilt inherent in being a Christian, all conspired to make Jill feel unsure and inadequate. Jill's "strong" husband, who incidentally played little role in nurturing the baby, tried to deal with his wife by blind reassurance initially, but gradually he withdrew from her and became impatient when she tried to voice her concerns. Jack would hold the baby at times, although he was afraid of showing physical affection and would never change or feed his son.

Jill started going back to church as a way of dealing with her distress; hence all these destructive messages were reinforced. Although her misery never reached the point of requiring psychiatric therapy, Jill did see her family doctor, who prescribed a minor tranquilizer. When the baby was fussy, Jill interpreted this as evidence that she was not a good mother; this would increase her guilt and the cycle would repeat itself. Unable throughout her life to develop a sense of competence in other areas, Jill was committed to playing "catch-up" in the maternal role and her need for positive strokes was insatiable. Jill relied on prayer a great deal; the more she prayed, the less she looked to her husband or her female friends for support. The couple's sexual relationship, which had never been very good, deteriorated further. During her good periods Jill would immerse herself in the baby to the exclusion of everything else; constantly preoccupied with Jake's health and safety, she could not be separated from him until he was almost one year old. When Jill was upset, her caretaking became inconsistent to the point of being chaotic at times.

When Jake first began taking an interest in feeding himself, Jill interpreted this to mean that she was not doing a good job feeding him herself and so she discouraged him. When he started crawling about she placed him in a playpen all the time for his safety. In doing this Jill was discouraging the boy's developing a sense of mastery of the environment and encouraging an overdependency on herself. This was made worse by Jill's punitive responses when her son would do something like tip over a glass accidentally. More and more the child retreated from any exploratory play and became withdrawn and passive; in the eyes of Jake's grandmother he was "a good little boy who didn't break things."

Because she was a good Christian, Jill "knew" it was wrong to be angry; in her verbal communications with her child and husband she tried to avoid any hint of anger or other emergency affects. When Jill's anger did break through, the anger/guilt cycle intensified. Her husband dealt with such feelings in a similar way. The child thus grew up in an atmosphere of pseudomutuality, full of incongruent communication, where what was said conformed neither with the tone of the voice in which it was spoken nor the parents' body language. Jake's own speech development was slow. He began being fearful of people and unwilling to approach them. (Social withdrawal is a common feature of schizophrenia.)

Perception, cognition, and speech development are closely interwoven. A child learns to think as he or she learns to interact verbally with adults who are communicating in a relatively congruent manner. If a child perceives that his mother is sad by looking at her eyes, all the while mother is smiling and chatting aimlessly, and if he is exposed to this kind of incongruent communication from both parents day after day, week after week, it is not difficult to see why disturbances of perception are so common in schizophrenics. If caretakers are incongruent communicators, as Christian indoctrination encourages people to be, the child may have problems in cognitive development. In particular, he may be unable to allow his thought processes to flow freely in a straight line. Loosening of associations is a common symptom of schizophrenia.

Jake's father's aloofness and his mother's inconsistency made it impossible for him to develop a basic trust in the world. He began to refuse to attend to his parents at all as a self-protective measure. This enraged Jake's mother, who relied on feedback from him for so much of her limited self-esteem. The family became an example of what Lidz would call a skewed family.

Anhedonia is another common feature of schizophrenia. As we have seen in earlier chapters, guilt about pleasure in favor of a commitment to suffering, in emulation of Jesus on the cross, is deeply embedded in Christian doctrine and liturgy. Since Jill was raised a Christian, and became a regular church goer early on in her child's life, this Christian anhedonic addiction to suffering was constantly being reinforced, especially in the sexual area. When Jake first began exploring his penis, his mother slapped his hand away. On the few occasions when the child did initially manifest pleasure in some activity, it was usually as an accompaniment to some motor activity such as banging a toy on the side of his playpen or, on rare occasions when Jake was let out of the playpen, trying to climb on a chair or stairs. On these occasions the activity, and the pleasure, would be cut short by Jill, who rationalized her behavior as a concern for her furniture, Jake's safety, or her "nerves." Since human interaction was so painful, and since pleasurable interaction with the inanimate environment was restricted, Jake became progressively withdrawn and less responsive.

The incongruent communication pattern that characterized Jake's family made it impossible for him to learn how to deal with the emotional side of life. Reduced emotional response and inappropriate emotional responses are part of the symptomatic picture of schizophrenia. The more Jake withdrew into himself, the more unhappy he became, and the more anxious and guilty Jill felt since she relied so much on Jake's happiness to make her feel good about herself as a mother. She was unaware of the conflict between her need to have a happy child and the manner in which her religious socialization tended to govern her interaction with him in a way as to make him anything but happy. Jill's guilt over her son's withdrawal and unhappiness made her more indulgent, more determined to prove she was a good mother by giving Jake what she thought he needed and even by trying to anticipate his needs. As time went by, Jake's individuation from Jill became severely compromised.

Jack, always on the sidelines, sensed vaguely that something was wrong but was unable to act in a way to change the situation. His own infantile needs, which had been fostered by his Christian upbringing and denied by his socialized macho male gender role, were completely frustrated. Sex was the only way in which he could make intimate contact with another human being and since his narrow view of sex combined with Jill's loss of sexual desire to shut that avenue off to him, Jack began to withdraw more and more from the family. His son became a competitor for his wife's affections, and therefore Jack's attitude toward his son became more and more rejecting. His dependency on his wife and his guilt concerning sexuality made it impossible for Jack to seek sexual satisfaction and affection outside his marriage.

A child who comes into the world with plenty of potential to adapt might be able to cope with this kind of early family environment without ultimately developing schizophrenia. Another child with only limited potential for adaptation, when exposed to such early experiences, may not become schizophrenic until adolescence or later, limping through the early developmental stages, barely coping with the adaptational challenges presented to him. However, when he has to cope with adult genital sexuality for the first time and when the ego defects make the establishment of any kind of adult relationship impossible, the clinical illness may emerge.

In discussing the relationship between culture and schizophrenia, H. P. Murphy has postulated that there are four main ways in which culture can affect the risk of developing schizophrenia:

1) the training or mistraining given regarding the processing of information

2) the complexity of information to which people are exposed

3) the degree to which decisions (acts or responses) are expected of all persons given complex or unclear information

4) the degree to which families prone to schizophrenia are discouraged from having or encouraged to have children.[9]

In terms of Murphy's formulations, there can be no doubt that throughout Jake's early life, he was mistrained in the processing of information, both that coming from inside himself and from the outside world. There was a complete incongruence between his emerging physical and emotional potential and the environmental response to it, a response that was chaotic rather than catalytic. The incongruent communication that characterized Jake's family made it extremely difficult for him to develop the cognitive emotional basis for further development. He had to learn to shape his behavior largely on the erratic moods of his mother rather than on a set of internal behavioral directives being elaborated within his own ego.

In the last few years there has been a resurgence of research interest in the role of family factors in influencing relapse rates in schizophrenia. Workers on both sides of the Atlantic have found that relapse is most likely to occur when patients return to families in which one significant relative, usually a parent, is emotionally overinvolved with, highly critical of, or overtly hostile to, the patient. The tendency of the family to induce guilt was found to be an additional predictor of relapse rates.[10,11] For some inexplicable reason, the unfortunate term "expressed emotion" is used to encompass these factors.

Some investigators in this field appear to bend over backward not to read etiology into this set of factors that have been found to be associated with relapse. This is so even when the factor has been found to be evident in the family for at least five years before the onset of the initial schizophrenic episode.[12] While one must always be wary of reading cause and effect into situations where one has noted only associations, workers in this field appear to show more than the usual amount of caution in this regard.

When one examines the approach usually taken to involve families of schizophrenics in treatment programs, the reasons for this extra caution become evident. Such programs often begin with a psychoeducational approach; as one group of researchers put it, there is an attempt to acquaint the family with the "current knowledge of the origins of schizophrenia, with care taken not to overtly or covertly implicate the family in the etiology or subsequent course of the illness."[13] In other words, the therapist/investigator, recognizing (or sensing) that the family is already feeling intense guilt about the sick member, tries to get their cooperation by starting with a strategy designed to allay that guilt. Regardless of the efficacy, not to mention the ethics, of such a strategy, its use does demonstrate how difficult it is for mental health professionals to deal with a family system in which guilt is so pronounced. Further, it is a measure of the power of guilt, so deeply engrained in Christian life, to dictate the behavioral responses of those professionals.

It seems reasonable to postulate an etiological significance for these family factors that appear to be causally related to relapse in schizophrenia. And on that basis let us examine these factors in light of what we have been saying throughout this book about Christian doctrine and mental health. The factor of emotional overinvolvement was really the subject of chapter 4 (dependency, interdependency, and self-actualization), although slightly different language was used. We have demonstrated that Christian teachings interfere with the process of "related individuation" and that a child who is under-individuated shows poor ego boundaries and runs the risk of remaining fused with or absorbed into the stronger organism, the parent. In order for this to be the case, the parent, whose individuation has also been severely compromised, would have to remain overinvolved in the life of the child.

Excess criticism and hostility toward the growing child also interfere with healthy adaptive growth, making it difficult for the child to feel good about himself. Negative attitudes toward the self which, as we have seen, are actually favored by Christian doctrine, lead naturally to negative attitudes toward others.

Schizophrenia may therefore be looked upon as a gross failure in ego integration, making adaptation to the various developmental stages difficult to impossible. The schizophrenogenicity of a Christian culture acts through the family to make it difficult for caretaking adults to be effective catalysts of their own offspring's growth processes.

MAJOR AFFECTIVE DISORDERS

A modern psychiatric textbook defines the affective disorders as "a group of clinical conditions, whose common and essential feature is a disturbance of mood accompanied by related cognitive, psychomotor, psychophysiological, and interpersonal difficulties."[14] It defines mood as "a pervasive or prevailing emotion that affects the total personality." The mood may be elevated in manic states in which the patient shows "expansiveness, flight of ideas, decreased sleep, heightened self-esteem, and grandiose ideas"; or it may be depressed, when the patient shows "loss of energy and interest, guilt feelings, difficulty in concentrating, loss of appetite, and thoughts of death or suicide."[15]

Classification of the depressive illnesses has, over the decades, reflected a variety of notions concerning etiology and phenomenology. "Neurotic" and "psychotic" were once considered useful distinctions. The terms "reactive" and "endogenous" were used when it was fashionable to consider that some depressions were due entirely to suprabiological precipitating factors while others, in which obvious precipitating factors were not immediately evident, were judged to be entirely biological in origin.

While confusion still surrounds the issue of classification, for those who still need to classify, it is useful to make the point that depression is a normal human emotion with which mentally healthy people cope in ways that do not result in the "cognitive, psychomotor, psychophysiological, and interpersonal" impairment. Many biologically oriented psychiatrists tend to dichotomize "normal" feelings of depression and the depressive disorders, preferring to view the latter as biological illness unrelated to emotional conflict or chronic use of maladaptive problem-solving strategies. It is difficult to understand what is gained by adopting this position other than high profits for the pharmaceutical industry, and the opportunity for some psychiatrists to distance themselves emotionally from their patients, to objectify them in a "we-they" fashion and thereby spare themselves the pain of recognizing that "there but for the grace of chance go I."

Whether an individual deals with depression in an adaptive manner or demonstrates the impairment that characterizes a depressive disorder appears to depend on two factors: the social support surrounding the individual and the individual's own ability to make use of such supports. One group of investigators puts it this way:

> Social support, instead of merely protecting an individual against the negative impact of stress, may itself be important in ameliorating depressive symptoms. Moreover, assuming that lack of perceived or actual social support is not just a manifestation of depression itself, our findings support the corollary that the lack of social support contributes to the creation of depressive symptoms.[16]

This is certainly borne out in the experience of couple and family therapists, who, whether or not they use drugs to help the patient symptomatically, are prepared to confront the real developmental and interpersonal problems that lie behind the "depression."

Samuel Novey goes so far as to state: "It is fundamental to modern psychiatry, however, that adequate interpersonal relationships are the bedrock of mental stability."[17]

We have, throughout this book, adduced evidence to show that Christian doctrine and Christian liturgy actually discourage the kind of human-to-human communication and negotiation skills that make for genuinely supportive human networks, the phenomenon of "Christian fellowship" notwithstanding. In a television broadcast on the subject of loneliness, evangelist Billy Graham beseeched his listeners to "come to Jesus Christ," thereby reinforcing the barriers that separate lonely people from their fellow human beings, those very barriers that Christianity has helped to erect.

If an individual has grown up with poor human relationship skills, his or her human support systems may not be or very effective, in which case full-blown clinical depression may emerge. This illness may show varying degrees of intensity and require a variety of psychiatric treatments; when it reaches the degree of intensity requiring mood-altering medication, we consider that we are then dealing with a major affective illness. The main classification system used today is: *bipolar disorder* (in which the mood disturbance is alternately one of mania and depression) and *unipolar disorder* (in which the mood is only one of depression).

ENVIRONMENTAL FACTORS IN AFFECTIVE ILLNESS

The search for *the* constellation of environmental, suprabiological factors operating in the etiology of depression has been as intensive as the quest for the Holy Grail, and about as productive. The main factors implicated along the way have been identified as personality factors, early maternal deprivation, loss of human supports associated with incomplete mourning, stressful life events that exceed the coping capacity of the individual, and learned helplessness.

Regarding the personality factors cited above, Kaplan and Sadock sum up the problem with these words: "It is widely believed that persons prone to depression are characterized by low self-esteem, strong superego, clinging and dependent interpersonal relations, and limited capacity for mature and enduring object relations."[18] As we have demonstrated throughout this book, these characteristics are inevitable products of the Christian belief system, one that preaches self-abasement as a means of ingratiating oneself with the deity, that discourages ego growth and innerdirectedness, and promotes superego growth and outerdirectedness with its reliance on external authority. The dependent, clinging relationship Christians are encouraged to develop with their God quite naturally becomes the paradigm for their relationships with each other in the absence of any training in how to make adult human relationships work.

Maternal deprivation is largely a direct result of the authoritarian pronatalist sex code operating in our society, which promotes the idea that motherhood is the only legitimate role for real women and which has encouraged women, even those who genuinely wanted children, to have more of them than they can care for emotionally or economically. Paul stated that childbirth was the only way in which women could be forgiven for the sins of Eve. By continuing to make it difficult for women and men to become knowledgeable about their sexuality, by continuing to resist the establishment of contraceptive and abortion services, many Christian denominations continue to contribute to unwanted pregnancies and maternal deprivation.

It is widely accepted that maternal deprivation, even to the point of child abuse, occurs in women who manifest an overt wish to have a baby. Closer examination usually reveals that such women have sustained severe narcissistic wounds which they are trying to heal by having a baby with whom they can identify in a narcissistic way—the "live doll" syndrome.

Being a competent mother is an adult activity and women can give *of* themselves *to* their babies only if they have been able to give *to* themselves without feeling guilt. A Christian society that promotes suffering as good for the soul, while it discourages adult self-esteem and human interdependency, is hardly an environment for encouraging women to develop their full potential as human beings; and if a woman has been socialized to ignore her own needs, how can she be expected to be sensitive to the needs of her infant?

The role of loss as a contributor to depression is a complex one. In fact, it is not the loss itself that appears to play an etiological role in depression but rather the way the loss is mourned. Christian attitudes toward death discourage healthy mourning in many ways, starting with the destructive impact of the resurrection myth. Since Jesus promised Christians a life after death, much of the message of "comfort" delivered at Christian funerals is geared to a denial of the very existence and permanence of death. A hymn common to the Anglican and United churches in Canada goes: "May we, whenever tempted to dejection, strongly recapture thoughts of resurrection. You gave us Jesus to defeat our sadness with Easter gladness." The essential Christian denial of death is illustrated in the famous hymn "Abide with Me"; here we find the words "Where is death's sting? Where, grave, thy victory? I triumph still, if thou abide with me."

Healthy mourning occurs when the bereaved is able to experience and express the full range of painful feelings mobilized by the loss of a loved one. Christian doctrine and practice encourage people to deal with such emergency emotions by beseeching "God" to take the painful feelings away, thereby making it difficult for human supports to sustain the mourner through these difficult times. It is often said at Christian funerals that "the widow was a real brick" or "he held up so well during it all." Denial of emergency emotions of all kinds is really encouraged in Christianity.

As background to a discussion of the role of stressful life events in the production of affective illness, we return to the issue of coping in the presence of anxiety (see chapter 4). Christian doctrine and liturgy have been shown to discourage the development of adult coping behaviors and the human-to-human relationship skills that enable people to cope in an adaptive way with the anxiety generated by stress.

The role of learned helplessness in depression has only recently come under scrutiny. It is now generally accepted[19] that children who, from an early age, live in a human environment that encourages them to develop mastery of their intra- and interpersonal environments, as well as the physical environment, are likely to develop a sense of competence and ultimately sound mental health. They are the adults who are more likely to cope with loss by allowing the mourning process to go forward naturally, and to adapt well to challenges and cope with stresses by use of their human support systems. These individuals are less likely to become depressed, having grown up with a lifelong sense of their own personal worth and competence, and an ability to trust in the human beings they cherish. By contrast, children who grow up influenced by Christian teachings develop a sense of powerlessness in the world, rather than a feeling of competence and mastery together with an inability to trust in the human support systems around them. It is logical that such individuals are more likely to grow up with a tendency to develop "clinical" depression when faced with loss or stress.

Christian doctrine promotes human helplessness by making it a virtue, indeed the sine qua non of a good Christian life. Paul said, "For when I am weak, then I am strong" (2 Cor. 12:10). A perusal of a common Anglican hymn book today will convince one that this is not simply an outmoded notion pushed by Paul, but is one constantly being reinforced: "Stand up! Stand up for Jesus! Stand in his strength alone; the arm of flesh will fail you; you dare not trust your own," and "Jesus Savior, pilot me over life's tempestuous sea." It is important to note that these lines explicitly discourage the development of personal mastery, warning that "the arm of flesh will fail you." They do not implore Jesus to help one find strength in oneself and human support systems to sail over "life's tempestuous seas." In order for a growing child not to be damaged by repeated exposure to such messages, he would have to be blessed with a considerably high level of innate adaptive capacity and with a familial and social environment that was able to neutralize the destructive impact of these messages.

CONCLUSION

In this chapter, I have tried to show how some of the more devastating teachings of Christianity might play a part in the genesis of schizophrenic and depressive disorders. This is an hypothesis I would like to see explored further by investigators in both these fields. However even those open-minded enough to admit the noxious effect of such deep-seated beliefs might nevertheless be unable to meet the methodological challenge posed by such an investigation. The messages about life that shape an individual's psychological, emotional, and physical growth come in so many forms, and at so many points in time, that finding the measurable variables would be like trying to catch a rainbow in a bottle. However, we can only hope that the methodological problem will ultimately be solved.

While the research strategies have not been developed to study the impact of Christian doctrine on individuals and families, the field of the psychology of religion has devoted considerable attention to the issue of "being religious." Much of this research is concerned with how the different ways of being religious correlate with other facets of life, notably mental health, racial tolerance, and concern for others.

There is a distinction between the thesis advanced in this book and the hypotheses tested by investigators in the field of psychology of religion. I am concerned with the overall impact of Christian doctrine on the individual in our society, whether or not the individual is now, or ever was, a card-carrying Christian. The non-churchgoer could have been compelled as a young child to attend church and Sunday school but given up religion as an adult, becoming an agnostic or atheist. Such an individual would be unlikely, however, to outgrow completely the effects of his early religious socialization; many of his behaviors and attitudes would have been formed at that time and remained unchanged, even though his cognitive, philosophical position had altered. The so-called believer could have remained or become a churchgoer and would be now considered "religious." In studies by researchers in the psychology of religion, he would be in the religious group while the non-churchgoer would be in the nonreligious group. I contend that the non-churchgoer and the "believer" would both be affected by Christian doctrine, the non-churchgoer probably less so, since the "believer," by attending church, would tend to get his religious ideas reinforced.

It is worth examining this research literature, however, since most of the studies were done on Christian subjects.

NOTES

1. Jules Henry, *Pathways to Madness* (London: Jonathan Cape, 1972), p. 374.

2. Roger J. Sullivan, "Psychotherapy: Whatever Became of Original Sin?" in Paul W. Sharkey, ed., *Philosophy, Religion and Psychotherapy* (Washington D.C.: University Press of America, 1982), p. 179.

3. Albert Ellis, "Is Religiosity Pathological?" *Free Inquiry* 18, no 2 (Spring 1988): 27–32.

4. Roy R. Grinker, Sr., "Neurosis, Psychosis, and the Borderline States," in Alfred M. Freedman, Harold I. Kaplan, and Benjamin J. Saddock, eds., *Comprehensive Textbook of Psychiatry* (Baltimore, Md.: The Williams and Wilkins Company, 1975), 1: 846.

5. Theodore Lidz, "Egocentric Cognitive Regression and the Family Setting of Schizophrenic Disorders," in Lyman C. Wynne, Rue L. Cromwell, and Steven Matthysse, eds., *The Nature of Schizophrenia: New Approaches to Research and Treatment* (New York: John Wylie and Sons, 1978), p. 528.

6. Louis A. Sass et al., "Parental Communication Deviance and Forms of Thinking in Male Schizophrenic Offspring," *Journal of Nervous and Mental Disease* 172, no. 9 (September 1984): 513–20.

7. Lidz, "Egocentric Cognitive Regression and the Family Setting of Schizophrenic Disorders," p. 528.

8. Lyman C. Wynne, "Methodologic and Conceptual Issues in the Study of Schizophrenics and Their Families," *Journal of Psychiatric Research* 6, suppl. 1 (1968): 185.

9. H. B. M. Murphy, "The Culture and Schizophrenia," in Ihsan al-Issa, ed., *Culture and Psychopathology* (Baltimore, Md.: University Park Press, 1982), p. 223.

152   Deadly Doctrine

10. Christine E. Vaughn et al., "Family Factors in Schizophrenic Relapse: Replication in California of British Research on Expressed Emotion," *Archives of General Psychiatry* 41 (December 1984): 1169.

10. Christine E. Vaughn et al., "Family Factors in Schizophrenic Relapse: Replication in California of British Research on Expressed Emotion," *Archives of General Psychiatry* 41 (December 1984): 1169.

11. Michael J. Goldstein and Jeri A. Doane, "Family Factors in the Onset, Course, and Treatment of Schizophrenic Spectrum Disorders: An Update of Current Research," *The Journal of Nervous and Mental Disease* 170, no. 11 (1982): 692–700.

12. Jeri A. Doane et al., "Parental Communication Deviance and Affective Style: Predictors of Subsequent Schizophrenia Spectrum Disorders in Vulnerable Adolescents," *Archives of General Psychiatry* 38 (June 1981): 679–85.

13. Goldstein and Doane, "Family Factors in the Onset, Course, and Treatment of Schizophrenic Spectrum Disorders," p. 687.

14. Harold I. Kaplan and Benjamin J. Sadock, *Modern Synopsis of Comprehensive Textbook of Psychiatry,* 4th ed. (Baltimore, Md.: Williams and Wilkins, 1985), p. 238.

15. Ibid., p. 239.

16. Carol S. Aneshensel and Jeffrey D. Stone, "Stress and Depression: A Test of the Buffering Model of Social Support," *Archives of General Psychiatry* 39 (December 1982): 1392.

17. Samuel Novey, "Considerations on Religion in Relation to Psychoanalysis and Psychotherapy," *Journal of Nervous and Mental Disease* 130 (1966): 316.

18. Kaplan and Sadock, *Modern Synopsis of Comprehensive Textbook of Psychiatry,* p. 244.

19. Martin E. P. Seligman, *Helplessness: On Depression, Development and Death* (San Francisco: W. H. Freedman & Co., 1975).

9

Christianity and Mental Health: The Research Findings

"No simplicity of mind, no obscurity of station can escape the universal duty of questioning all that we believe."
—W. K. Clifford[1]

"My son, be not curious, nor trouble thyself with idle cares."
—Thomas à Kempis[2]

The correlation of "being religious" with being "something else" (mentally healthy, prejudiced, or concerned about others) does not "prove" cause and effect. If, for example, a study demonstrates that people who are religious in a certain way are also mentally healthy or unhealthy, we cannot say for sure that either state caused the other. Each could be the result of a third variable not yet identified. Also, most of the studies in this area are based on self-report, paper and pencil questionnaires which do not always take into account the social desirability factor, the human tendency to want to respond in a way that makes one look good, however inaccurate the response. On the other hand, some studies do not rely simply on what the individual subject says about his or her attitudes but on measures of the individual's behavior.

In 1982, Batson and Ventis published a rich, in-depth review of all of the literature bearing on this subject, and it is their work that is summarized in this chapter. They examined the various ways of being religious and correlated them with mental health, prejudice, and concern for others. Their definition of religion is a broad one: "whatever we as individuals do to come to grips personally with the questions that confront us because we are aware that we and others like us are alive and that we will die. Such questions we shall call existential questions."[3] This definition differs significantly from most others, specifically the one used throughout this book, namely, that religion "is that system of beliefs that looks to divine supernatural forces for the meaning of human existence and for the rules of behavior designed to cope with existential anxieties." As pointed out in chapter 2, Batson and Ventis's broad definition of religion makes "religion" as a distinct concept disappear almost entirely. Confronting existential questions is not in itself a religious activity; accepting prepackaged, ready-made answers to those existential questions which invoke a supernatural divine being, is.

So complete has been the religious takeover of our language in this area that not only has the word "moral" been almost completely co-opted by god-talkers, but this search for meaning and a preoccupation with existential questions has been mislabeled as a religious activity. There are good reasons for this. Until recently, religion was the only philosophical and educational game in town, to the point where we still have several universities with the designations "Catholic," "Lutheran," "Baptist," and so on. Another historical reason why the search for meaning and a preoccupation with existential questions has been labeled as "religious" is that there were certain pressures operating to encourage people to come up with religious answers. Academic interest in the historical Jesus, for example, is little more than two hundred years old; the nineteenth century was a time of considerable and scholarly ferment in this area.[4] Given this, it may be no exaggeration to say that the impact of Christian doctrine, with its addiction to absolutism, is the main stumbling block to the development of educational programs that might awaken children's minds to a healthy, liberating, mind-expanding exploration of existential questions.

Drawing on the pioneering work of Gordon Allport and Bernard Spilka and their respective associates,[5,6] Batson and Ventis postulated three ways of being religious: a means orientation, an end orientation, and a quest orientation. The means orientation is akin to the extrinsic orientation of Allport and Ross,[7] and is concerned with the degree to which one uses religion as a means to other, self-serving ends—social, political, and economic. The person with the means orientation goes to church because he or she feels it is good to be seen there. Concerns about eternal verities play little role in their religious life.

The end orientation is akin to the intrinsic orientation of Allport and Ross; those who score high on this orientation are devout in their adherence to religious beliefs and practices, and view religion as central to life—indeed, the way to finding meaning in life.

Earlier on in chapter 2, we questioned the sharp distinction between these two orientations, on the grounds that people with the end orientation were as motivated by self-interest as were those with a means orientation. The means-oriented person is concerned about this life; someone with an end orientation has his eye on eternal rewards. Hence there is a powerful element of "means" in the "end" orientation.

The "quest" orientation has been described by Batson and Ventis as "an approach that involves honestly facing existential questions in all their complexity, while resisting clear-cut, pat answers."[8] It is defined as "more psychologically adaptive" than the other two methods.[9]

Central to most definitions of religion is a supernatural being or god; and the question of meaning in life is always intimately bound up with that divine personage. Batson and Ventis have made the definition of religion so broad that it clearly encompasses both atheists and theists, religionists and humanists. In their quest orientation, they are clearly talking about people who are not "religious" at all by most definitions of religion. In fact, people with the quest orientation are clearly those with a truly scientific approach to life. Anyone who honestly faces "existential questions in all their complexity while resisting clear-cut, pat answers" is a scientific humanist through and through. Religion, by contrast, normally presumes a need for, and a reliance on, "clearcut, pat answers." Hence Batson and Ventis are essentially comparing two ways of being religious (means and end) to what is essentially a scientific approach to life.

Science itself is not concerned solely with the physical world and with events, things, and processes that can be counted and measured; research is only one aspect of being scientific. Indeed, many people engaged in research are not really scientific at all, in that they do not approach their data with an open, questioning, mind but rather seek to use the science of statistics to buttress their biases. Being scientific in one's approach to life is an attitude regarding all aspects of life that extends even to facing existential questions for which there are not, and may never be, "clear-cut, pat answers." Science cannot be advanced if all such existential questions, for which no research design has been developed, are ignored or relegated to the category of "being religious." We will return to this topic at the end of the chapter.

RELIGION AND MENTAL HEALTH

In examining the ways of being religious and the issue of mental health, Batson and Ventis had to deal with a large number of studies using varying definitions of mental health: (1) absence of mental illness, (2) appropriate social behavior, (3) freedom from worry and guilt, (4) personal competence and control, (5) self-acceptance or self-actualization, (6) personality unification and organization, and (7) open-mindedness and flexibility. Most of the studies defined mental health in terms that fit definitions 3, 4, 5, and 7. Few studies defined mental health in terms of definition 1, 2, and 6.

Batson and Ventis, after examining in detail fifty-seven studies, came to the following conclusion: the means orientation to religion had "a rather pervasive negative relationship" to mental health *regardless of how mental health is conceived.* In other words, people who are religious for short-term social rewards are not very mentally healthy when measured by these characteristics: freedom from worry and guilt, personal competence and control, self-acceptance or self-actualization, and open-mindedness and flexibility.

When it came to examining the end orientation to religion, Batson and Ventis found that it was positively associated with greater freedom from worry and guilt, as well as enhanced personal competence and control, but not with greater open-mindedness and flexibility. As the authors point out, the greater "personal competence and control" were based on reliance on God, not on oneself. In other words, it was not really a personal competence but a blind reliance on the omniscience and omnipotence of the deity. This combination of apparent freedom from worry or guilt, combined with an apparent sense of personal competence that is really a reliance on God, coupled with a lack of open-mindedness and flexibility, is actually a definition of smugness, a quality especially characteristic of the "born again" Christian.

The quest orientation which is, as discussed earlier, more a scientific than a religious attitude toward life, was discovered to be associated with a high level of personal competence and control based on self-reliance, not on reliance on God. It was also associated with greater open-mindedness and flexibility than was the end orientation. However, it was not associated with greater freedom from worry or guilt. As Batson and Ventis put it: "The intrinsic end orientation leads to freedom from existential concerns and a sense of competence based on one's connectedness to the Almighty, but at the same time an inflexible bondage to the beliefs. In contrast, the quest orientation leads to neither."[10]

The association of greater worry and guilt in the quest orientation by comparison with the end orientation deserves some comment. Many people with a questing, nonreligious approach to life were born into a religious family and somewhere along the way rejected their religious orientation or, more properly, grew beyond the need for such an orientation. However, Christian indoctrination runs deep; therefore, it is not surprising that people subjected to such indoctrination would still be feeling its effects in later years. This is especially true since, in rejecting the religious orientation in favor of a scientific questing orientation, they also rejected the placebos offered by organized Christianity, such as confession and being "saved."

The social desirability factor most certainly operates here as well. Christians are not supposed to feel guilty if the guilt has been washed away by the blood of Jesus, so there is a marked tendency for Christians to deny guilt even when it is clearly operating in their lives and helping to shape their behavior. Many Christians lead restrictive, austere, pleasure-free lives, as a way of minimizing the opportunities for guilt to arise. The more religious the individual, the more guilt is denied, a finding that any sensitive psychotherapist will confirm. Hence Christians, when answering a questionnaire, are likely to show the same degree of denial that they demonstrate in the clinical situation. By contrast, people with a quest orientation to life have no such need to deny any guilt they may feel; it is more acceptable for them to be open and honest.

The finding of greater open-mindedness and flexibility in those with a questing, scientific orientation than in those with a religious orientation agrees with our own argument throughout this book. The price religious people have to pay for the existential nostrums offered by Christianity is to have a straitjacket placed on their human potential. Many Christians, especially those engaged in scientific pursuits, try to deny that this is the case; they even talk about science as being a gift from God to enable humans to conquer the earth and subdue it as the Bible instructs. Some Christians claim to be scientific about some areas of life, but even for them a truly scientific approach to the totality of human existence is impossible; it would be too painful emotionally for them to turn their telescopes and microscopes on the human need for a sustaining deity, and on the strategies used by religious institutions to keep that need alive in human beings.

The gist of all this is that being religious is quite definitely not associated with greater mental health when compared to a scientific, questing approach to life. The latter approach's association with more "worry and guilt" is probably traceable, in large part, to early Christian socialization and to a lesser need to deny emergency emotions. But even if this is the case, surely this is a small price to pay for the greater "open-mindedness and flexibility" that characterizes the quest orientation.

RELIGION AND RACIAL PREJUDICE

Turning away from the issue of mental health, the relationship between being religious and racial intolerance is one that has preoccupied students of the psychology of religion since 1946, when Allport and Kramer found that white American Protestant and Catholic students were more likely than those with no religious affiliation to be prejudiced against blacks.[11] Batson and Ventis, reviewing forty-four studies earried out since 1946, found that thirty-four of these showed "a positive relationship between amount of prejudice and amount of interest in, involvement in, or adherence to, religion."[12] Eight studies, mostly from northern states, showed no relation and two studies showed a negative relationship; interestingly, these two final studies were on pre-adolescents and adolescents, suggesting that the longer one remained associated with the Christian church, the more likely one was to become prejudiced. Batson and Ventis comment on the statistical significance of their conclusions: "If one were to compute the probability of obtaining evidence this strong for the positive relationship between being religious and being more prejudiced when such a relationship really did not exist, it would not be noticeably different from your chances of winning the Irish sweepstakes—provided you had never entered."[13]

When the issue of racial prejudice was examined in relation to the two ways of being religious (means and end), it was discovered that those with a means orientation were highly prejudiced, while those with an end orientation exhibited a level of prejudice closer to those with a questing, scientific approach to life. However, few studies done after 1946 made allowances for the element of social desirability.* In a series of experiments in which behavioral measures of prejudice were introduced, the authors found that apparent differences between the two ways of being religious were indeed a function of social desirability. When it came time to act in accordance with the attitudes they claim to have on paper (for example, by choosing a black or white subject to interview), those with an end orientation showed a degree of prejudice similar to that shown by people with a means orientation.

Subjects with a questing, scientific orientation to life scored low on prejudice even when the element of social desirability was controlled. As for the two religious orientations, Batson and Ventis sum up their results in this way: "Being religious in one way, as an extrinsic means, seemed to relate to increased prejudice even when social desirability was controlled. Being religious in another way, as an intrinsic end, related to self-reports of decreased prejudice, but when social desirability was controlled, the relationship disappeared."[14]

These findings raise interesting questions. Why, when Christianity is supposed to be a religion of love, are Christians more intolerant of those who do not have the same skin color? In South Africa, white Christians even seek and—not surprisingly—find biblical support for the suppression of their black Christian brethren. The question may be asked another way: Why are those who have grown beyond the need for the comfort of the Christian religion, or who were minimally exposed to it, more racially tolerant than

---

*Social desirability is that characteristic prompting people to answer questionnaires in a way that makes them look good, rather than in a completely truthful manner. This is why behavioral measures—what people actually do under certain circumstances—are usually more revealing than self-report questionnaires.

those who are still believers? Is there something about the doctrine of the Christian church that tends to make people seek and find scapegoats?

The answer to this question is undoubtedly a resounding yes. An individual burdened with as much guilt as a Christian is encouraged to bear would, if he or she does not become completely psychotic, have to externalize some of the self-hatred which characterizes the true Christian. Scapegoats for that hatred have never been hard to find.

RELIGION AND CONCERN FOR OTHERS

With the discovery that people who are religious Christians may be less mentally healthy and more racially prejudiced than those who are not religious, a third question comes to mind: Do Christians really show more concern for their fellow creatures? Batson and Ventis reviewed seven studies of self-report questionnaires which demonstrated that religious people were more helpful than nonreligious people. However, when they examined five studies that used behavioral measures of helpfulness rather than self-report questionnaires, they found that there was no correlation between degrees of religiousness and helpfulness. In other words, when the factor of social desirability was removed, religious people were no more or less helpful than nonreligious ones.

A study by Darley and Batson,[15] modeled after the Good Samaritan story, turned out to be particularly revealing. Theological students were tested to see what determined whether or not they would stop on their way to class to help someone in obvious distress. It turned out that religious orientation did not seem to determine their behavior. Rather, it was more a question of how rushed students were to get to their class. However, among those who did stop, there was a distinct difference in one aspect of helping behavior between those with an end orientation and those with the quest orientation. The person taking the role of a sick derelict lying in the doorway of a building was instructed to insist that he could manage on his own and did not need the student to do anything. Those with a quest orientation respected his wishes more than those with an end orientation. The latter group appeared to have an internal need to help that overrode their ability to be sensitive to what the other person really needed.

It appears from all this that Christians can associate themselves with projects that give them a sense of being good Christians, when the helping is not on an interpersonal level, and when they are not required to tailor their help to the real needs of a human situation. Otherwise, Christians are no more helpful than nonreligious people; indeed, if the Darley and Batson study is measuring a real dimension, Christians are more insensitive since they tailor all their efforts to their need to ingratiate themselves with the deity. In their book *The Long Dying of Baby Andrew,*[16] Robert and Peggy Stinson described their experiences with the medical staff with whom they had contact during the tragic circumstances surrounding the birth and eventual death of their premature infant. It was their experience that non-Catholic doctors, especially non-Christian doctors, were more responsive to patients' concerns and feelings than were the strongly Catholic physicians, who insisted on following their own rigid religious program.

CONCLUSION

It is safe to conclude that committed Christians, when compared to those with a more scientific approach to life, do not fare very well when it comes to mental health, racial prejudice, and concern for others. On self-report, Christians appear less beset with worry and guilt than nonreligious people; however, the psychological mechanism of denial and the need to give socially desirable answers may account for this difference. They appear to manifest as much personal competence and control as those with a scientific questing orientation; but this, too, is spurious, for it is not a real sense of personal competence but rather a reliance on an omnipotent deity. Committed Christians show more racial prejudice than those with a humanist orientation, while in interpersonal situations they are no more helpful than nonbelievers. Indeed, Christians may be less so, since they are insensitive to the real needs of the person in distress as they persist in acting according to their Christian belief system. Summing up their research, Batson and Ventis conclude: "This evidence suggests that religion is a negative force in human life, one we would be better off without."[17]

Batson and Ventis's definition of religion and their inclusion of the questing, existential approach to life among ways of "being religious" require one final comment. Most researchers in the field of the psychology of religion work in universities and schools or faculties of religious studies. Many are believers themselves, and their "scientific" work is undoubtedly biased by their belief system. Many others in the field, while not believers themselves, are still working in a discipline where believers, many of them masquerading as people with a true quest orientation, continue to hold the political power. Reading Batson and Ventis's illuminating book, one must conclude that their evidence supports the conclusion that religious people are less mentally healthy, more prejudiced, and less sensitive in interpersonal situations than are nonbelievers.

Stated as bluntly as this, such a finding would not go down very well in religious "academic" circles. It is possible, therefore, that Batson and Ventis were motivated by political considerations both in their choice of a definition of religion that clearly embraces the nonreligious, atheistic, humanist orientation, and in their discussion of the questing, existential scientific approach to life as if it were one other religious orientation. If this supposition is correct, namely, that Batson and Ventis deliberately couched their findings in ways that would placate believers, we have one more piece of evidence supporting the all-pervading power of the Christian church in our society.

NOTES

1. W. K. Clifford, "The Ethics of Belief," in Gordon Stein, ed., *An Anthology of Atheism* (Buffalo, N.Y.: Prometheus Books, 1980), p. 280.

2. Thomas à Kempis, *The Imitation of Christ* (Chicago: Moody Press, 1980), p. 183.

3. C. Daniel Batson and W. Larry Ventis, *The Religious Experience* (New York: Oxford University Press, 1982), p. 7.

4. R. Joseph Hoffmann, "Biblical Criticism and Its Discontents," *Free Inquiry* (Fall 1982): 17–21.

5. G. W. Allport, *The Individual and His Religion* (New York: Macmillan, 1950).

6. R. O. Allen and B. Spilka, "Committed and Consensual Religion: A Specification of Religious-Prejudice Relationships," *Journal for the Scientific Study of Religion* 6 (1967): 191–206.

7. G. W. Allport and J. M. Ross, "Personal Religious Orientation and Prejudice," *Journal of Personality and Social Psychology* 5 (1967): 432–43.

8. Batson and Ventis, *The Religious Experience*, pp. 149–50.

9. Ibid., p. 170.

10. Ibid., p. 249.

11. G. W. Allport and B. M. Kramer, "Some Roots of Prejudice," *Journal of Psychology* 22 (1946): 9–30.

12. Batson and Ventis, *The Religious Experience*, p. 257.

13. Ibid., p. 257.

14. Ibid., p. 281.

15. J. M. Darley and C. D. Batson, " 'From Jerusalem to Jericho': A Study of Situational and Dispositional Variables in Helping Behavior," *Journal of Personality and Social Psychology* 27 (1973): 100–108.

16. Robert and Peggy Stinson, *The Long Dying of Baby Andrew* (Boston: Little, Brown and Company, 1983).

17. Batson and Ventis, *The Religious Experience*, p. 306

10

Christianity and Health Care

"If thou wilt make any progress in godliness, keep thyself in the fear of God, and desire not too much liberty. Restrain all thy senses under the severity of discipline, and give not thyself over to foolish mirth"

—Thomas à Kempis[1]

"Psychological health, to a large extent, consists of being in touch with one's feelings, and to believe that one is not morally permitted to experience certain feelings is to declare war on one's emotions."

—George H. Smith[2]

CHRISTIANITY VERSUS PSYCHOTHERAPY

Many attempts have been made to draw parallels between the counseling of the Christian cleric or counselor and the practice of psychotherapy.[3] One writer even goes so far as to make the bizarre claim, "Psychologists and theologians are concerned with the same issue in their attempts to extract meaning from an existence which is constantly evolving."[4] But as we have learned from our study of Christian belief systems, the committed Christian does not "extract" meaning from existence; instead, he spends much time and energy trying to impose on his surroundings a specific world view. If there are similarities between Christian "pastoral" counseling and psychotherapy, they are not substantive; in a long list of fundamental issues, the two approaches are based on diametrically opposite views of the human animal and the human condition.

163

While there are many schools of psychotherapy, psychotherapy itself may be broadly defined as a "talking treatment" in which trained therapists help patients or clients to uncover conflicts lying beneath their symptoms and to find more adaptive ways of dealing with those conflicts, as well as any other conflicts that emerge as treatment progresses.

Robert Sabga has invented a very useful term, "religious detoxification," to describe an educational/therapeutic process designed to help people throw off the destructive myths, attitudes, and behavior patterns produced by religious socialization and to grow beyond the need for such noxious sources of "comfort."[5] Sabga's experience working in drug treatment centers made him appreciate the parallel between addiction to drugs like alcohol or tobacco and the addiction to harmful belief systems. Whether it is a toxic chemical or a toxic belief, the process of weaning is similarly painful and difficult. Although psychotherapists rarely confront patients' religious belief systems directly, a comparison of the values underlying the process of psychotherapy with those underlying Christianity demonstrates that in effect psychotherapy is a form of religious detoxification.

As we have seen in chapter 3, Christian doctrine and liturgy promote an orientation away from self-understanding and toward God. Psychotherapy, by contrast, encourages an understanding of self as the sine qua non of the therapeutic process. And while Christianity encourages self-loathing as a strategy for incurring favor with God, a strategy that unfortunately finds its way into human interactions, psychotherapy encourages self-esteem and self-love on the grounds that these are necessary prerequisites to esteem and love of others.

As Edmund D. Cohen has pointed out (see chapter 2), Christianity, fosters dissociation within the individual, chiefly through its emphasis on the perpetual state of war between the "flesh" and the "spirit," but also through such strategies as the promotion of guilt over normal human feelings and impulses. Psychotherapy tends to promote harmony among the various levels of human functioning: affective, cognitive, biological, behavioral, and verbal. It aims to help people feel at home with themselves.

In the verbal area, for example, Christians are discouraged from developing congruent communication patterns with other people. The internal dissociation inculcated by Christian teaching makes this difficult in any case; but Christians are actively encouraged to distrust their fellow human beings, particularly nonbelievers, and to trust in God instead and to communicate only with Him. Psychotherapy, whether individual, conjoint marital, family or group therapy, works to the extent that patients are able to improve their communication skills. As this happens, more trust develops, better negotiation patterns emerge, and the human-to-human support system grows stronger. The better the human support group, the less attraction there is to god-talk.

As we saw in chapter 5, Christianity, with its emphasis on original sin and the sacrifice of Christ on the cross, relies heavily on the promotion and manipulation of guilt as leverage for exerting control over the lives of men and women. But while guilt, especially over sex, may bring about some shallow behavioral conformity and superficial acceptance of certain attitudes, it is the primary enemy of adaptive human behavior. The main task of the psychotherapist in this case is to help patients act less out of reflex guilt and more from their own appreciation of their needs and wants, so that they may lead more responsible and productive lives.

RELIGIOUS STATUS EXAMINATION

In psychiatry, the "mental status examination" is a crucial component of a complete psychiatric appraisal during which the interviewer seeks to evaluate the patient's mental functioning in all its aspects, including memory, presence or absence of thought disorders (e.g., delusions or hallucinations), and computing ability. No candidate for professional certification in psychiatry can approach his or her final examinations without being proficient in conducting an examination of this type.

Surprisingly, given the necessity of evaluating so many other areas of the mental state, health professionals generally, including mental health professionals, still commonly avoid asking patients and clients questions about sex and religion. To the casual outsider this must be somewhat bewildering, since out sexuality and belief systems play so important a role in the formation of our psyche and outlook on life. To make up for this curious omission, Helen Singer Kaplan has proposed the inclusion of a sexual status examination as part of the routine psychiatric appraisal and has spelled out what information should be obtained.[6]

Health care professionals avoid the issue of religion and the role it plays in patients' suffering even more stringently than the sexual area. As one researcher puts it, "It seems that clients must virtually stand on their head to get the therapists to even inquire about their religious convictions, much less examine them! Questions regarding the consistency, credibility, coherence, and internal consistency—let alone motivating power—of religious convictions are gingerly passed over."[7]

The naive notion that religion has no negative effect on mental health can no longer be tolerated. It is time, then, to consider the development of a "religious status examination" in the training of health care workers. Such an examination of patients in our Christian society would be a logical extension of the mental status examination; it would explore the degree to which patients still accept the psychotic world view of Christianity, Eric Fromm's *folie à millions*. And since Christian doctrine can have a definite impact even on individuals who no longer claim to be religious, such an examination would have to go beyond the stated religiosity or religious affiliation of the individual.[8]

What follows is not meant to be a definitive example of a religious status examination, but rather some of the key points that should be touched upon in such an examination. If the patient does believe in God, how does he or she perceive that personage? As benign or benevolent? As jealous, capricious, vengeful, or loving? How does the patient relate to Christian teachings about humility, self-denial, and self-abasement? Does the individual think it is against God's wishes for human beings to love themselves, to be assertive in trying to get their needs met? Does God want us to suffer as Christ suffered? What should we feel guilty about? How have Christian teachings about sexuality and reproduction affected the individual? How much of the Christian belief system does the individual accept, and have patients' own thinking about Christian doctrine and teachings affected how they live their lives? In other words, to what extent have they lived an unexamined life, and to what extent have they been prepared to question?

If patients have been able to question the religious beliefs of their childhood, how far along the road from believer to free thinker have they come? Although they may have intellectually given up dogmatic Christian beliefs, is there evidence that some of these beliefs still affect their attitudes and behavior?

PSYCHOTHERAPY OF THE RELIGIOUS PATIENT

Writers on this topic oten emphasize that therapists need to "respect" the religious views of the patient or client, views that are often referred to as "spiritual values"; although what form that "respect" should take and how the therapy should proceed in the light of this "respect" on the part of the therapist is never made clear.

If we refer to Robert Sabga's model of religious detoxification and view addiction to a religious belief system as we would an addiction to alcohol or tobacco, we can discern how to proceed with religious patients seeking psychotherapy. In dealing with the nicotine or alcohol addict who is not motivated to get over the addiction, a direct confrontation in the form of a recommendation to stop smoking or drinking is usually not effective. Refraining from doing so does not represent the physician's "respect" for the addiction, but rather a "respect" for the strength of the addiction and the tenacity with which the patient asserts his or her twisted autonomy by resisting any pressure from outside to change, notwithstanding the fact that such addicts are anything but autonomous in the face of the addiction. There should even be room in all of this for respect for the patient's "right" to remain addicted.

While a physician may decide not to waste time and energy trying to persuade the patient to stop smoking or drinking, it is the physician's responsibility to make sure that the patient knows all about the deleterious consequences of the addiction; in addition, the physician should be prepared to treat the treatable consequences of that addiction, such as heart disease, liver cirrhosis, or lung cancer. When it comes to psychotherapy of the religous patient or client, it is equally futile for the therapist to try to get the individual to renounce an addiction to god-talk; in fact, such proselytizing is foreign to psychotherapy. However, it is incumbent on the therapist to make the patient aware of those aspects of his or her particular belief system that run counter to the mutually agreed upon goals of the therapy. It the patient avoids working in therapy because of a belief that everything is in God's hands anyway, that belief must be challenged in the light of the fact that the patient has come for the kind of help that requires his or her active participation. If a man uses his relationship to God as a wall between himself and other members of the family, it is important for the therapist to be explicit in pointing this out. While it is inappropriate to attempt to undermine a patient's belief in God, it is important to demonstrate how a patient's individual, at times idiosyncratic, views about God contribute to the problems for which he or she is seeking psychotherapeutic help.

After a successful course of therapy, a patient or client may come to modify some of the more destructive aspects of the religious addiction, but continue to embrace a vague theistic belief. Or the patient may progress to the point where theism has lost all appeal and so reject god-talk outright. It could be argued that relinquishing a need for the supernatural is evidence of truly adaptive human behavior and that the patient is not "cured" until this takes place. However, the goal of psychotherapy is not to produce freethinking atheists, any more than it is the goal of education is to produce Nobel laureates or of physical fitness programs to spawn Olympic athletes. The orientation to god-talk runs deep in our society, and the current direction of our educational systems does not give one much encouragement to believe that the situation is likely to change very soon.

CHRISTIANITY AND GENERAL HEALTH CARE

In chapter 1 illness behavior, i.e., the individual's overall response to symptoms, was seen to be largely determined by lessons learned early in life about illness and suffering. Given the evidence advanced in this book regarding the role of Christian doctrine in encouraging suffering, a religious status examination should be as important to the general physician as it is to the psychiatrist, if not more so. Most, though by no means all, patients who present to the psychiatrist have accepted that their problem is something outside the biomedical arena and has something to do with problems in living rather than lesion illness. At the level of general medical care, the office of the general practitioner, many of the forces shaping patients' help-seeking behavior encourage both patients and doctors to interpret the problem purely on a biological/medical level. The patient is treated simply as a machine; there is little or no effort to integrate the physical with the emotional and the psychological.

Indeed, the structure and organization of the health care system as it relates to physicians, the main actors in the health care drama, encourage a rigid biomedical view of suffering. For one thing, doctors are not rewarded for keeping people healthy, but for tending them after they have become ill. The so-called fee-for-service system in which physicians are remunerated for patient visits and thereby encouraged to see as many patients as possible, limits the amount of time a phsycian can spend with any one patient to explore all the factors contributing to his or her suffering. This is so, even if the doctor does have an inclination to explore intrapersonal, interpersonal, or social sources for an individual's pain. And physicians who do try to get away from assembly line medicine to explore patients' problems in depth, usually find that their income suffers considerably.

The power of the international pharmaceutical industry is certainly an important factor in all this. The more superficial physicians are in dealing with patients, the more likely their interventions will include the prescription of some form of medication. Chlordiazepoxide (Valium), a so-called minor tranquilizer, became the most widely prescribed drug in the United States as early as 1972. One student of the drug industry reports that profits from worldwide sales of this tranquilizer are worth roughly one hundred million dollars annually, and that in Canada its price was twenty times the total production cost.[9] And this was before passage of the Canadian government's Bill C-22, which removed many of the existing regulations governing the pharmaceutical industry.

Nineteenth-century medicine, with its emphasis on the disease (lesion illness) model, still has a powerful hold on the minds of those in charge of medical education. Newer innovative models of medical education, while conceptually refreshing, have not lived up to their promise and have had little impact on the total situation. One reason is that graduates of such programs end up having to contend with a traditional health care system; the shape of their practices is determined largely by economic forces over which they have no direct control.

The nineteenth-century disease model of illness still holds sway for other reasons as well. While physicians vary a great deal in terms of their readiness to explore deeper explanations for patients' suffering, regrettably, most prefer to make the often totally unwarranted assumption that such suffering is lesion-related. In this way they are able to maintain a detached attitude ("me doctor, you patient"). Once the physician and the patient move to deeper levels of problem solving, the patient's conflicted relationships with parents, spouse, or boss may turn out to be related to his suffering; in this event, the "me doctor, you patient" stance must make way for a different approach. If physicians wish to be helpful at this point, they must be able to empathize with the patient by recognizing the conflicts with important authority figures in their own lives.

But what has all this to do with Christianity?

Many physicians are either religious themselves or are still very much affected by the fallout from Christianity's emphasis on the human-to-god bond over the human-to-human bond. Hence this band-aid brand of medicine allows them to remain at a comfortable distance from their patients and their human problems.

The disease interpretation of illness is also attractive to the suffering patient, in whom no lesion exists. The infant in all of us likes simple solutions to our problems, and the one characteristic of adulthood that is most difficult to achieve is the readiness to accept the complexity of most of life's problems. Individuals with an infantile approach to life are more likely to nourish the hope, even the expectation, that simple remedies for their suffering are available; doctors often encourage this expectation by ordering a long list of unnecessary tests looking for the lesion, the demon of the medical exorcist. Just as children magically expect a mother's kiss to cure any problem, so do patients expect a magic pill to make them feel better, thus enabling them to avoid confronting deeper issues in their lives.

The Christian church may have lost the battle to dictate how human beings must interpret events in the physical world, although the so-called "creation scientists" are reluctant to admit defeat in this area. The more important battle has yet to be joined, however—the struggle for the human "mind." The fact that health care professionals have not been encouraged to examine the potentially noxious impact of Christian doctrine on their patients and that our educational systems are reluctant to turn the light of unfettered human inquiry on the phenomenon of religion itself, are indicators of the power Christianity still holds over our society.

One strategy used by the Christian church in its relentless pursuit of power in the blatant appropriation of every new liberating trend in human society and every new insight into human behavior, accompanied by massive "advertising" campaigns designed to convince people that the church itself was responsible for the innovation. This at times frantic struggle to achieve relevance has often led to bizarre distortions of basic Christian doctrine. Such distortions are the subject of the next chapter.

NOTES

1. Thomas à Kempis, *The Imitation of Christ* (Chicago: Moody Press, 1980), p. 65.

2. George H. Smith, *Atheism: The Case against God* (Buffalo, N.Y.: Prometheus Books, 1979), p. 323.

3. E. Mark Stern, ed., *Psychotherapy and the Religiously Committed Patient* (New York: The Haworth Press, Inc., 1985).

4. Joseph. E. Morris, "Theology and Psychology: A Humanistic Perspective," in Paul W. Sharkey, ed., *Philosophy, Religion and Psychotherapy* (Washington, D.C.: University Press of America, 1982), p. 161.

5. Robert Sabga, "What is Religious Detoxification?" medium II, Erindale College, Toronto, October 5, 1983, p. 5.

6. Helen Singer Kaplan, ed., *The Evaluation of Sexual Disorders* (New York. Bruner-Mazel, 1983).

7. Samuel M. Natale, "Confrontation and the Religious Beliefs of a Client," in *Psychotherapy and the Religiously Committed Patient,* p. 108.

8. The degree of *folie* can, of course, vary. Albert Ellis has concluded from his work in psychotherapy that adherents to the more absolutist and perfectionist groups are likely to be more frequently and intensely disturbed than those whose religious views are more liberal. See Albert Ellis, "Do Some Religious Beliefs Help Create Emotional Disturbance?" *Psychotherapy in Private Practice* (Winter 1986): 106.

9. Joel Lexchin, *The Real Pushers* (Vancouver: New Star Books, 1984), p. 19.

11

Christian Double-Think and Newspeak

"When the Christian 'reformer' comes forward to declare that sex is not evil and that sex outside of marriage may, after all, be permissible—and when he calls on Christian Churches to spearhead his new movement—one must wonder if it ever occurs to him that he is 19 centuries too late."

—George H. Smith[1]

"Whatever was true now was true from everlasting to everlasting. It was quite simple. All that was needed was an unending series of victories over your own memory. 'Reality control ' they called it: in Newspeak, 'double-think.' "

—George Orwell[2]

Winston Smith, the hero of George Orwell's futuristic novel, *Nineteen Eighty-Four,* had a peculiar job in the Ministry of Truth. He was one of thousands of workers whose task was to rewrite history according to current party policy. If, in a speech, Big Brother made a prediction that did not come true, all records of that portion of the speech—in newspapers, books, pamphlets, and film—had to be erased and substituted with a revisionist account making it look as if Big Brother had correctly predicted events. If a former political alliance of Oceania with Eurasia threatened to become an embarrassment to Big Brother, all accounts of that alliance had to be eradicated from the public record. This process was politely called "rectification." In this way, "all history became a palimpsest, scraped clean and reinscribed exactly as often as was necessary."[3]

For the average Christian, God is portrayed, like Big Brother, as unchanging, steadfast, omnipotent, and omniscient—as it says in Psalm 100, "His truth endureth to all generations." However, a close examination of the record shows that God changes his mind a lot; in fact, quite a lot.

Coupled with the myth of the unchanging deity is the equally tenacious fiction that Christianity has played a role in civilizing and humanizing society; in fact, the influence has been in the opposite direction. The Christian religion has maintained and extended its power by appropriating ideas from the wider human culture: from science, especially behavioral science; freethinkers; humanists; and, more recently, feminists, all the while taking the credit for the change. Bertrand Russell has commented on this phenomenon in this way: "It is amusing to hear the modern Christian telling you how mild and rationalistic Christianity really is, and ignoring the fact that all its mildness and rationalism is due to the teaching of men who in their own day were persecuted by all orthodox Christians."[4]

Let us now look at some broad areas in which the Christian church has sought to "humanize" itself by assimilating certain civilizing trends. However, each time the church steals an idea or makes a move in a humanistic direction, it creates a conflict with the traditional teachings arising out of core doctrine.

CHRISTIAN FELLOWSHIP

In the early life of the church, vows of silence were fostered as a way of promoting union with God; but such imposed silence works against the development of bonds between people. In fact, "not talking" to each other (sometimes called "sulking"), is one of the best causes *and indices* of a dysfunctional relationship. Thomas à Kempis's *The Imitation of Christ* contains over twenty explicit statements warning the faithful to avoid the company of their fellows. To take one example: "Thou oughtest to be so dead to such affections of beloved friends, that, as much as concerns thee, thou shouldest wish to be without all company of men. Man approacheth so much the nearer unto God, the further off he departeth from all earthly consolation."[5] Is it too extreme to suggest that admonitions such as these contribute to the innumerable problems in human relationships we see at all levels from the marital dyad to relationships between nations?

However, vows of silence, and social and geographical isolation gradually gave way to a modified human support group, one that could be controlled and channelled along "Christian" lines—hence Christian fellowship.

CHRISTIANITY AND MORALITY

Morality is another area where religions generally, and Christianity in particular, are all too ready to take credit where none is due. In fact, for many people the idea that morality comes from religious indoctrination is so strong that for them, "morality" and "religion" are almost synonymous terms. Yet all the facts point to the probability that where religion is unchallenged by the wider culture, as in the case of medieval Christianity and certain conservative Islamic states today, we see a virtual reign of terror. There is certainly nothing moral about the Inquisition, the witch hunts, or the religious police in Islamic states. George H. Smith goes so far as to state: "Any link between religion and morality is not only unjustified, it is enormously harmful. The religious view of morality is still widely accepted; children are raised by it and men attempt to live by it—with the result that millions of people practice, in the name of morality, what amounts to emotional and intellectual suicide."[6] Ludwig Feuerbach put it even more strongly: "Wherever morality is based on theology, wherever the right is made dependent on divine authority, the most immoral, unjust, infamous things can be justified and established. . . . If morality has no foundation in itself, there is no inherent necessity for morality; morality is then surrendered to the groundless arbitrariness of religion."[7]

CHRISTIANITY AND WAR

War is another area where the church has incorporated attitudes from society at large and made them her own. Until quite late in the present century, God was portrayed as a God of war; the Crusades represented a glorious phase in the history of Christendom. A few centuries ago, Holy Wars were viewed as they are currently by Islam; the message, explicit in hoth Islam and Christianity, was that if you lost your life in war (the ultimate human obscenity), you were sure of a place in heaven. Martin Luther once wrote: "No one need think that the world cannot he ruled without blood. The civil sword can and must be red and bloody."[8] In the latter part of the nineteenth century, the Vatican had an army in the field defending the papal states against the Italian unification forces. In 1870, the pope's army was defeated and the territory owned by the Vatican shrank from approximately one third of the Italian "boot" to what is now Vatican city. As time went by, God became perceived more and more in peaceful terms. Now that he no longer has an army to command, the pope, the Vicar of Christ, has become the Prince of Peace. As Charles W. Sutherland has written: "Bereft of military power, the church naturally became less bellicose, which partially explains its new consistency in preaching a morality of peace."[9]

CHRISTIANITY AND DEMOCRACY

Whenever the pope travels he makes headlines speaking and praying, not only for peace but for democracy and "freedom," although he fails to mention that such freedom does not include the freedom to think for oneself, to regulate one's reproductivity, or to express oneself sexually in ways proscribed by church teaching. As for democracy, it is an open secret that the Roman Catholic Church has been the implacable foe of that fragile human institution since its birth, becoming a reluctant supporter only when the great powers containing millions of Roman Catholics became democracies, at least in name. Currently, dissenting Roman Catholics, clerical and lay, in that most democratic country, the United States, are causing the Holy Father the most distress. Those who have been lulled into believing that the Catholic Church has always been the champion of democracy should read the *Syllabus of Errors,* the 1864 pronouncement of Pope Pius IX which condemned free speech and the principle of religious toleration.

Nor is there any reason to believe that the respect for democracy goes very deep in Protestantism. The so-called religious right in the United States would have no qualms whatever about abolishing democracy if it had (or gets) the power to do so. In 1988, a fundamentalist TV evangelist actively sought for the Republican nomination for president. Lawrence Lader, in his book *Politics, Power and the Church,* has documented the determined efforts of the Catholic-Fundamentalist alliance, during the favorable climate of the Reagan presidency, to destroy the American Constitution's First Amendment guaranteeing separation of church and state, and to establish a Christian theocracy.[10]

CHRISTIANITY AND RELIGIOUS TOLERANCE

Perhaps the most startling shift in church policy was the recent message from the pope titled "If You Want Peace, Respect the Conscience of Every Person." In this 6,000 word document the head of the Roman Catholic Church made some astounding statements to the effect that, "People must not attempt to impose their own 'truth' on others." The pontiff defended "the inalienable right to follow one's conscience and to profess and practice one's own faith."[11] The 1864 *Syllabus of Errors* severely condemned religious tolerance in the Roman Catholic Church; in the 1990s, we witness a complete volte-face. If this represents a change in God's will, how sad that God did not change his mind before the Inquisition, before all those pogroms against the Jews, and before all those brave missionaries got themselves killed spreading the Christian message all over the globe. In reality, this new open-mindedness represents nothing but a political maneuver on the part of the pope. Since Christianity is now the largest religion numerically on earth, the church may find it politic to be less hard-nosed.

The obvious conclusion to draw from the Church's shifting its social positions is that the unchangeable God of War somehow metamorphosed into the God of peace, that he also changed his mind about slavery and other political institutions—in short, that the angry God became a just God. At each juncture, experts in theology—the Winston Smiths of Ecclesiastica—had to make the scriptural record fit the current policy. In doing so, they were able to make people almost forget that the God of Peace had once been a God of War, that the Christian Church was at best a reluctant ally of democracy, and that it had once officially countenanced slavery. However, it will require a lot of Orwellian "rectification" before Christianity's addiction to proselytization will be affected by the pope's message urging respect for other people's religious views.

But if the theologians of previous generations were kept busy trying to convince everyone that this capricious God was really unchanging, omnipotent, and omniscient, they did not have to work at the pace of their modern counterparts. The god experts of the 1990s are faced with overwhelming evidence from modern behavioral science, humanism, and feminism demonstrating the anti-human nature of Christian doctrine and teachings. No distortion of reality is too bizarre in Christianity's struggle to appear relevant to today's world. American Catholic priest and sociologist Andrew Greely, writing in the *New York Times,* has claimed that the popular family sitcoms on TV are really Christian morality plays in which Christian family living is portrayed, even though religion is noticeably absent from most of them.

CHRISTIANITY AND SEXUALITY

It is in the area of human sexuality and gender roles that Christian double-think and newspeak become most bizarre. We saw in chapter 6 how Christianity promotes sexual ignorance and pronatalism. Within the past few decades, many Christians have become aware that traditional church teachings about sexuality have been largely responsible for the crisis in population growth, not to mention much personal suffering on the part of millions of couples and individuals. A number of denominations have changed their policies on a wide range of sexual and reproductive issues, such as contraception, abortion, and homosexuality.

Every time the church lurches reluctantly and convulsively to try to keep up with the culture at large, the theologians scurry to find obscure scriptural footnotes they can use to justify the shift. At a recent pastoral conference on sexuality and spirituality,[13] one Catholic theologian gave this ecclesiastical version of Orwellian rectification the pretentious title of "Retrieval Critique Analysis." In so doing, she admitted that there were "compelling examples of how the bible [*sic*] and our historical theological reflection have themselves participated in and actively promoted dualistic ways of thinking and acting." She further admitted that "in its many historical, political, and institutional forms, the Church has often been a source or cause of distortion and alienation." The solution, therefore, "seeks to remember and restore the life-giving and liberating message in the bible." This along suggests a revisionist attitude.

Another attempt to undo the damage done by centuries of Christian emphasis on the war between flesh and spirit is the new "embodiment theology." A Protestant theologian at the same conference admitted that "the ancient dualistic split between man and woman, continue to wreak their havoc." He pleaded for a host of new embodiment theologies, including "erotic theologies" to replace the old dualistic one. He admitted that Christian tradition has given religious sanction to homophobia, which in turn thrived on "erotophobia" (see chapter 6). The theologian further acknowledged that the Christian church has been "the main institutional legitimizer of compulsory heterosexuality," adding that "sexuality's power was feared, restrained, and disciplined."

Another theologian postulated a "paradigm shift" in Christian thinking concerning human sexuality. The old dualistic paradigm, with which sex therapists are only too familiar, is another term for what we have called the coercive pronatalist sex code (chapter 6), which is noted for being profoundly sexist, anti-pleasure, and anti-human. He proposed a new "holistic paradigm," corresponding to what we have called the humanist neutronatalist sex code (see chapter 12). This theologian neglected, however, to acknowledge his debt to secular humanism and behavioral science; intellectual honesty and academic courtesy are apparently not requirements of "retrieval critique analysis" or "embodiment theology." Instead, he proclaimed that the "radicality" of this new paradigm stems in part from "seeds planted long ago." Insisting that the Church "is not having to foresake its past so much as draw on different strands that have been long ignored or denied validity," he made the astounding assertion that the new paradigm was "in part the child of the old." It is very difficult to understand how anyone's credulity could be stretched far enough to see any connection between this new "holistic paradigm" and the old "dualistic paradigm." Even Big Brother would not be happy with this shoddy example of rectification.

But let us assume for a moment that this theologian is correct in his new interpretation of God's holy will regarding sexuality, thus displacing the pronatalist sex code of St. Paul and St. Augustine. This leads one to the astounding conclusion that for over sixteen centuries, Christian clerics have relentlessly promoted teaching on sexuality that was really *not* what God intended for his people. How can these theologians remain so sanguine about all this? Why did God let the clergy operate for almost two millennia promoting false beliefs that caused such harm to the people God is supposed to love so much? Did God not know what was going on? Could it be that God really is the vicious, capricious sadist that is depicted in many parts of the Old and New Testaments? Or is he a political pragmatist who changes his mind whenever the nonbelieving opposition puts enough pressure on his human spokespersons to get them to alter his policy—of course through a process of "retrieval critique analysis"—insisting that he had been saying this all along to people who weren't listening?

In the field of what is called "feminist theology," another revisionist approach was taken, to the effect that the doctrine and teachings of the Christian church have really not contributed to the oppression of women. The fly leaf of *Sexism and God-Talk,* by theologian Rosemary Radford Ruether, summarizes the book's feminist revisionist approach: "By carefully examining the root teachings of the Bible and the writings of ancient goddess-oriented cultures, Ruether brilliantly envisions a new, nonsexist understanding of Christianity." These "root teachings" consist of finding feminine characteristics in the depiction of God in parts of the Old Testament and in the parables of Jesus where men and women appear to be treated equally.[14] This brings to mind a crude analogy, that of a Jew joining the Nazi party in the hope of getting the party to reverse its position on anti-Semitism. Mary Daly, a Catholic theologian who made a valiant attempt to find a place for women within the fold of the Roman Catholic Church, was finally forced to conclude that "sexism was inherent in the symbol system of Christianity itself and that a primary function of Christianity in Western culture has been to legitimize sexism."[15]

CHRISTIANITY AND SELF-ESTEEM

In chapter 3, we saw how important self-esteem is in the development of a healthy personality. We also saw how traditional Christian doctrine worked against the growth of self-esteem in people exposed to it. An awareness of this fact has seeped into the consciousness, and possibly the conscience, of some Christian god-talkers, who perhaps dimly realize that telling people they are sinners does not make them feel very good about themselves, and may even lead them to behave accordingly. Even televangelists, using the language of modern behavioral science, are now promoting self-esteem for Christians. One of their pat phrases is "A strong ego but not a wrong ego," with the claim that there is such a thing as "holy pride." One popular TV evangelist writes that "self-esteem and self-respect represent a healthy pride in ourselves as God's loved and redeemed creation."[16] This is not healthy self-esteem but rather a reformulated justification for Christians to continue hiding their feelings of self-loathing behind an arrogant mask of condescension toward anyone who does not share their views.

In his book *Fragmented Gods,* sociologist Reginald Bibby documents the declining fortunes of the Christian churches in Canada. A compelling reason for this, he argues, is that "Religion has frequently been associated with the denunciation of self. Christianity, for example, in both its Roman Catholic and Protestant expressions, has not lacked for emphasis on human sinfulness, the need to deny self, the importance of being poor in spirit, the acknowledgement of one being capable of nothing apart from God."[17] Professor Bibby's advice to the modern Canadian church is that it literally reverse its sixteen-hundred-year-old precedent, and start promoting self-love and the intrinsic worth and potential of the individual human being.

In a book titled *Why Christians Break Down,*[18] William A. Miller, a Christian minister, points to the church's "tendency to express a kind of false personal security and goodness by denying and repressing the dark sides of human personality." Miller also cites the "oppressive demands made by the Church in terms of behavioral expectations" as well as its tendency "to paint much of life as either black or white with little consideration for the specific situation. . . . The Church has seemed to stress the worthlessness of man, seemingly encouraging people to be ashamed of themselves almost to the exclusion of being proud of themselves."

The author, a hospital chaplain, wrote this book in the naive hope that he could influence the church to humanize itself in order to eliminate or at least reduce these harmful "tendencies." Reverend Miller thereby joined a large group of like-minded Christians who have recognized how anti-human and destructive Christian teachings and doctrines are. What they all fail to realize, however, is that these malignant tendencies are inherent in the core doctrine of the Christian Church, and that band-aids, such as "retrieval critique analysis" and "embodiment theologies," are no cure for doctrinal cancer. As George H. Smith has pointed out, "If such theologians were truly concerned with man's happiness on earth, they would begin by repudiating, totally and unequivocally, Christianity itself."[19]

No amount of reinterpretive whitewash can cover up the essential feature of Christian doctrine, the one that separates it from all other modern religions—namely, the crucifixion/resurrection myth. If someone does not subscribe to that myth, it is difficult to understand how he or she could claim the label "Christian."

The crucifixion/resurrection myth makes no sense unless the doctrine of original sin is invoked to explain why Christ's death on the cross was necessary. No matter how much "joy" a Christian is supposed to experience when contemplating this "wondrous gift," the bottom line is that his or her innate sinfulness drove God to this extreme. While the "born again" Christian is washed free of the taint of original sin by the blood of the Lamb, he can never expiate this deep-seated guilt that must go with being Christian. This "ground-in guilt" is not meant to be washed away, since it constitutes the main source of the priest's or minister's power.

Pity the poor Christian! Not only must he suffer the effects of the dehumanizing Christian doctrine itself, but, with the seemingly endless number of Christian denominations and sects, must also contend with the conflicting versions of that doctrine. Now a third source of conflict has arisen. Should Christians believe in the traditional God or in the laundered, whitewashed version promoted by the Retrieveal Critique analyst? The Bible is full of references to God as a vengeful, vindictive deity who is capable of meting out the most hideous punishments to those who disobey Him; yet at the same time, modern Christians are supposed to believe in the God of "Love" and "Mercy," whose retributive hand may be stayed if one submits body and soul, heart and mind, to him. However, even this is not absolutely certain. God is peddled as a God of peace, yet popular hymns like "Onward Christian Soldiers, Marching us to War" proclaim the Church of God as moving "like a mighty army" led by "Christ/Master," whose followers go "forward in battle." One well-known Christian denomination is the Salvation Army, whose members adopt military ranks.

One of the advantages Big Brother had over his theological counterpart was that, in Oceania, the old record could be obliterated totally. In Christianity the old record remains in place for all to see, making the task of Christian rectifiers all the more difficult. Feminist theologians would love to erase St. Paul's first epistle to Timothy, in which Eve is blamed for the transgression in the Garden of Eden, thus sentencing women throughout time to salvation only through child bearing "if they continue in faith and charity and holiness with sobriety."

The modern Christian may sigh with relief listening to a sermon on "embodiment theology" and the new "holistic paradigm" reqarding human sexuality. One can only wonder about the reaction if the following lesson is this: "For to be carnally minded is death; but to be spiritually minded is life and peace. Because the carnal mind is enmity against God; for it is not subject to the law of God, neither indeed can be. So then they that are in the flesh cannot please God" (Rom. 8:6–8).

Christianity survived the Renaissance. It survived the Inquisition, the Crusades, the Borgia popes, and the Holocaust, and it shows every sign of surviving the antics of Jimmy and Tammy Bakker and Jimmy Swaggart. So long as the messages of Christianity remain unchallenged in society and in the educational systems in the Western world, it will continue to thrive.

180   Deadly Doctrine

The challenge, if it comes, must of necessity come from humanism, which is the subject of our final chapter.

NOTES

1. George H. Smith, *Atheism: The Case against God* (Buffalo, N.Y.: Prometheus Books, 1979), p. 309.
2. George Orwell, *Ninteen Eighty-Four* (London: Penguin Books, 1984), p. 34.
3. Ibid., p. 39.
4. Bertrand Russell, *Why I Am Not a Christian* (London: Allen and Unwin, 1967), p. 35.
5. Thomas à Kempis, *The Imitation of Christ* (Chicago: Moody Press, 1980), pp. 219-20.
6. Smith, *Atheism: The Case against God,* p. 304.
7. Ludwig Feuerbach, *The Essence of Christianity,* trans. George Eliot (Buffalo, N.Y.: Prometheus Books, 1989), p. 274.
8. Martin Luther, *Werke* 15: 302, quoted in *The Great Quotations,* compiled by George Seldes (Secaucus, N.J.: The Citadel Press, 1983).
9. Charles W. Sutherland, *Disciples of Destruction* (Buffalo, N.Y.: Prometheus Books, 1987), p. 211.
10. Lawrence Lader, *Politics, Power and the Church* (New York: Macmillan, 1987).
11. *The Toronto Star,* December 19, 1990.
12. Andrew Greely, *The New York Times,* reprint the (Hamilton, Ontario) *Spectator,* August 1, 1987.
13. "Sexuality/Spirituality," special issue of the *SIECCAN [Sex Information and Education Council of Canada] Journal* 2, no. 2 (Summer 1987).
14. Rosemary Radford Ruether, *Sexism and God-Talk* (Boston: Beacon Press, 1983).
15. Mary Daly, *The Church and the Second Sex* (Boston: Beacon Press, 1985), p. 17.
16. Robert H. Schuller, *The Be (Happy) Attidudes* (New York: Bantam Books, 1985), p. 39.
17. Reginald W. Bibby, *Fragmented Gods* (Toronto: Irwin Publishing, 1987), p. 263.
18. William A. Miller, *Why Christians Break Down* (Minneapolis, Minn.: Augsburg Publishing House, 1973).
19. Smith, *Atheism: The Case against God,* p. 309.

12

The Future: Homo Religiosus
or Homo Sapiens?

"It is possible that mankind is on the threshold of a Golden Age: but, if so, it will be necessary first to slay the dragon that guards the door, and that dragon is religion."

—Bertrand Russell[1]

"One thing that has become evident is the need to emphasize new directions for humanism."

—Paul Kurtz[2]

The designation Homo sapiens (wise man), applied to our species at this stage of our cultural evolution, is a misnomer. Religious indoctrination of children is still tolerated, if not encouraged, by the state; people are building new Christian churches rather than turning existing ones into museums. TV evangelists amass huge fortunes by open extortion in the name of Christ; surely, a more accurate term is Homo religiosus (religious man).

Whether Homo religiosus will evolve into Homo sapiens in time to prevent the species from extinction, is becoming increasingly unlikely. Having obeyed God's instruction to multiply and subdue the earth, we now find that, in carrying out His Holy Will, we may have irrevocably damaged the environment required to sustain all forms of life. The Roman Catholic Church, although unable to prevent members of its flock from using family planning and abortion services when these are available, is able to exert sufficient pressure on Catholic legislators throughout the world, to block the establishment of enough such programs to defuse the population bomb.[3]

But in order to end this book on a positive note, let us assume that the outlook is not altogether hopeless. In the words of the poet T. S. Elliott, "for us there is only the trying."[4]

Not to state the case too strongly, indoctrination with the core doctrine and other teachings of the Christian Church constitutes a form of mental and emotional abuse. The attitudes generated by Christian teachings are deeply embedded in the structure of society and in the psyches of its individual members. In the area of gender role socialization, feminists have made us painfully aware of the depth and extent of attitudes that are not only anti-female but anti-human, and they have called upon us all to grow beyond our reflex sexism. A similar kind of in-depth desensitization is called for in other areas of life shaped by Christian doctrine, such as pleasure and guilt, sexuality and reproduction, interpersonal communication, expression of human emotions, self-actualization, and self-esteem. Even if (letting imagination run riot) all Christian god-talkers from the pope down were to repudiate the entire belief system tomorrow, the situation would not suddenly change. The attitudes run too deep for that to happen.

Bertrand Russell states that we should slay the dragon guarding the threshold of humanity's future; perhaps we should instead encourage the dragon to die a natural death by making it impossible for him to continue feeding on human gullibility. This will come only through a process of education, which can unlock the doors of the religious prison we have built to help us cope with our existential angst. Many prisoners of religion would like to be sprung loose; in order for this to happen, it must become more widely known that religion is not the only existential game in town. The other one is humanism.

In order to understand what humanism is (or, more properly, what a humanist is), we should contrast a humanist with a Christian. The Christian depicted here best fits the fundamentalist or Roman Catholic mold, but on many levels he is found among the more "liberal" denominations as well.

Humanists rely on human supports. Christians are encouraged to place their reliance on a supernatural agent or deity.

Humanists affirm that this life is to be lived to the fullest. For Christians, this life is to be lived in a manner designed to please this supernatural being who will then reward the supplicant with life everlasting.

Humanists declare that the meaning of life is what we put into it. Christians believe that the meaning of life is determined by God's will as described in the scriptures, and interpreted by his human agents.

For humanists, human reason is the only meaningful basis for determining moral behavior. For Christians, moral behavior consists in following a set of rules derived from God as determined by some of his mortal agents.

Humanists accept the scientific approach to aquisition of knowledge in all areas of life; Christians accept the scientific approach to life in all areas *except* those that threaten their system of beliefs, which must be accepted on faith.

Humanists acknowledge that guilt-free pleasure is the raw material of sound personality growth. Christians are not meant to enjoy themselves too much in this world, but are encouraged to keep their eyes on the rewards of the next.

Humanists are encouraged to accept all feelings as natural and to make a distinction between feelings and behavior. Christians are taught to be suspicious and fearful of many of their feelings, such as anger, which is one of the seven deadly sins. And for the Christian, there is no distinction between feelings and behavior. According to St. Paul, "He that looketh after a woman to lust after her hath already committed adultery in his heart."

Humanists support the equality of the sexes. Christians have been socialized to view women as inferior to men.

Humanists may be quite vocal in criticizing supernatural beliefs, but are tolerant of individual believers who are really victims of their addictive belief systems. Christians make little distinction between belief and believer; historically Christianity has persecuted and massacred nonbelievers.

Humanists are encouraged to like themselves, to esteem themselves as worthwhile individuals, on the grounds that if one cannot like oneself, one cannot like anyone else. Christians are encouraged to consider this as pride and to believe that one must abase oneself in order to find favor with God.

Humanists believe in the essential goodness of human beings. Christians believe that human beings are "fallen," and that all true goodness resides in God, to whom we all should grovel in order to bask, vicariously, in this goodness.

Humanists try to live with ambivalence, ambiguity, and uncertainty, dealing with existential angst by reliance on each other. Christians cannot deal with uncertainty; they look for support in faith in the deity and his unerring design for the universe.

Humanists stress that nothing can be outside the realm of free inquiry and are prepared to question everything, including their own cherished beliefs. For Christians many beliefs are beyond question, and must be accepted on faith.

Humanists want their children to learn to think critically and to grow according to their own lights into unique human beings. Christians want their children to be indoctrinated into becoming perfect models of what a Christian should be.

HUMANISM VERSUS RELIGION IN EDUCATION

Christians justify their establishment of religious schools on the "grounds" that the public school system has been heavily infused (or, in their minds, infected) with humanistic beliefs. Nothing, however, could be further from the truth. Although the public schools, if they do their job properly, teach children how to think, they are very careful not to encourage them to think too critically about their religious beliefs, nor about social attitudes toward life derived from religious beliefs. However, to the god-talkers, a child who is encouraged to think at all is a loose cannon; he or she might start using human reason to ask questions about religion. Hence the need to establish their own schools in order to create a "learning" environment that places developing young human minds in doctrinal straitjackets.

Notwithstanding the existence of religious "schools" and "universities," the Christian church has, since the Renaissance, been the implacable foe of true education. The current campaign to reassert the literal interpretation of the Genesis creation myth as "Truth" is a case in point; and a measure of Christian desperation is the absurd oxymoron "creation science."

However, even in nonconfessional public schools, where hymn singing, Bible reading, and praying are completely absent, the Christian presence is still felt. In Alberta, a Christian public high school teacher was able, for many years, to use his classroom as a platform from which he could spew his anti-Semitic view of history. The man was eventually charged as a hate monger in a court of law and found guilty. However, the real culprit in this case was not this teacher but the Alberta Ministry of Education and the local school board for allowing these racist views to go unchallenged under the guise of education. Had this teacher been the educator he was paid to be, he would have made sure that competing views were presented to his students so that they could come to their own conclusions; and the school board should have made certain that this happened.[5]

The best evidence of the fact that humanism does not control the public education system is the lack of *real education* about religion in the public school curriculum. One teacher with the courage to try something in this area was actually dismissed from his job. He had shown his students a documentry film on Christian fundamentalism and then given them an assignment to interview people in their families on the role religion played in their lives. The furor was so intense and so immediate that the local school board ordered a cancellation of the student project and suspended the teacher. The mere act of asking people to use their human intelligence to examine their religious beliefs and the real impact of those beliefs on their lives, was simply too threatening.[6]

Why should we not educate children about the role of religion in human affairs throughout history, just as we educate them, or try to, about so many other aspects of life? The reason is simple. Having resisted vigorously all attempts by human reason to shed light on matters it has considered its prerogative from the Renaissance onwards, Christianity would resist even more forcefully any attempt to shine the light of reason on Christianity itself. Christians everywhere agitate for more "religious education" in the schools, by which they mean "religious indoctrination"; except in some circles, true education about religions is unheard of. It is safe to say that the humanist alternative will be alive and well only when our educational systems can critically examine the claims that religion promotes moral human behavior, that Christ died for our sins, that the traditional Christian attitudes about sexuality and reproduction come from God, and that God has reserved for us a place in heaven if only we accept what the Christian snake oil salesmen tell us.

The public educational systems of the so-called Christian countries ought to be opening up the growing child's mind about the real role of religion throughout human history. And they should also be helping to prepare the adults of tomorrow for the job of cleaning up the mess left by centuries of Christianity's oppressive influence on education, notably in the area of sexuality and interpersonal communication.

HUMANISM AND SEXUALITY

Christian opposition has largely prevented the establishment of truly effective, enlightened sex education programs. While some schools deal with this subject on a superficial level, their programs are usually mounted out of negative motivations, such as preventing AIDS or unwanted pregnancy, rather than out of a real desire to help children learn how to get guilt-free pleasure from this area of their lives. Moreover, schools are usually most circumspect in their treatment of the subject lest they offend Christian sensibilities. Few of them have been able to deal with the myths generated by Christian teachings which have been shown to lie at the root of so many adult sexual problems— myths concerning masturbation, noncoital behaviors and homosexuality, and male and female sexual roles.

Even when the goal is a modest one of preventing unwanted pregnancy, the system fails; as Stevi Jackson puts it, "If one reason for sex education is to prevent unwanted pregnancy, would it not be helpful to tell girls about the sensual potential of their bodies, and to let boys and girls know that it is possible to give and receive sexual pleasure without engaging in the act of intercourse?"[7] Currently some young people do engage in petting to orgasm, but this is usually viewed as "kid stuff" and merely a prelude to the "real thing." When passion overrides the preaching, young people are conditioned to think "intercourse," all too often without any means of protection against pregnancy or venereal disease.

In chapters 6 and 7 we saw how the authoritarian pronatalist sex code, derived largely from Christian teachings about sexuality, was shown to be a major factor in promoting sexual dysfunction. Over the past century a new code has been slowly emerging, one that might be called a humanist neutro-natalist sex code. it is called humanist since it does not rely on secular or ecclesiastical authority to define the rules of sexual behavior, but rather encourages enlightened individuals and couples to take charge of their own sexual and reproductive lives. such a code is neutronatalist since it neither promotes nor discourges births.

In chapter 6, we discussed the various characteristics of the pronatalist sex code; what follows here is a similar breakdown of the humanist neutro-natalist sex code to show how it contrasts with the authoritarian and repressive pronatalist sex code.

Sexual Enlightenment

The humanist sex code promotes enlightenment about sexuality on the grounds that knowledge is power in this as in all areas of human existence. Such knowledge enables people to exercise their sexual and reproductive options.

Sexual Awareness in Childhood and Adolescence

The humanist code assumes that children need to be encouraged to accept their emerging sexuality as it manifests itself subjectively in feelings of primitive arousal, or objectively in terms of wet dreams, breast development, and menarche. Such open acceptance is an essential component of integrative personality growth, which helps to equip children with the means of protecting themselves from sexually predatory adults.

Sensual and Sexual Pleasure

The humanist code recognizes the important role played by sensual pleasure through the medium of touching and caressing, both for its own sake and as a necessary precursor to, and integral component of, healthy, normal sexual pleasure. While currently there is some social sanction for females to develop this capacity, through their experience in nursing infants, there is still a tendency for males to separate their sensual from their sexual needs or to indulge themselves only insofar as the experience leads to genital sex, specifically intercourse.

The humanist code promotes the view that sexual pleasure for both sexes is a part of healthy, normal, sexual experience, provided it occur in a non-exploitative relationship.

Sexual Behaviors and Orientations

The humanist code accepts as natural the total range of sexual behaviors and orientations, provided that decisions are well informed (i.e., considering the risk of AIDS in unprotected anal intercourse) and socially responsible (preventing unwanted pregnancy), and provided that negotiation between equal participants in nonexploitative, open, and honest.

Parenthood

The humanist code recognizes the legitimacy of voluntary nonparenthood on the grounds that parenting is too important a social role to be forced on anyone; and just as not everyone is qualified to be a symphony conductor, a plumber, or a politician, so not everyone may be cut out to be a parent. This code also recognizes the rights of the individual and the couple to regulate reproductivity preconceptively, through contraception, as well as postconceptively, through abortion.

Responsibility for Sexual Behavior

The sexual enlightenment advocated by the humanist code emphasizes that individuals will be in a position, and indeed expected, to accept full responsibility for their sexual behavior. They will not be able to resort to such religiously biased excuses as the doctrine of "irresistible impulse" or "The devil made me do it," or explain away male aggression against women by arguing, "She was only asking for it."

Gender Role Socialization

Under the humanist sex code, individuals are encouraged to develop to the fullest all of their potential as human beings, unhampered by rigid, archaic, gender roles that have been shown to be detrimental to both personal development and harmonious relationships.

Sexual Exploitation

The humanist neutronatalist sex code rejects all forms of sexual exploitation of human beings, whether that be in the form of social and political pressure to reproduce or (as in modern China) not to reproduce; interpersonal exploitation ("You'd have intercourse with me if you really loved me"); or commercial exploitation ("You'll be real popular with the girls or boys if you buy this car, this nail polish, or this shampoo").

HUMANISM AND HUMAN COMMUNICATION

The influence of Christianity, preoccupied as it is with one-way communication to God, is also demonstrated by the failure of schools to teach children the basic principles of two-way, human-to-human communication and negotiation. One specific example of the need for such education is the difficulty of expressing such emergency emotions as anger, which, as we saw in chapter 4, is a problem area for many people.

We need to recognize the contribution of Christianity to our stunted, warped attitudes about anger, as we are doing slowly in the area of sexuality. When we do so, we can develop educational programs aimed at helping children to learn adaptive responses to feelings of anger, which relieve the pressure in the individual being affected, do not hurt the person whose behavior is the object of the anger, and possibly improve the relationship. Before dismissing this notion as fanciful, we would be wise to consider that much of the work of psychotherapists is devoted to helping people to accept their feelings as natural and to give up maladaptive strategies for coping with anger which are self-destructive and damaging to relationships. If these attitudes and behavior patterns can be modified *therapeutically* during adult life, it will be more humane—not to mention cost-effective—to develop educational programs designed to prevent the formation of destructive behavior patterns in young children.

Already some schools have programs for helping children use their innate intelligence to help them learn about ethical and moral behavior. Situations are described which require discussion of the ethical decisions to be made, and to which the child applies his or her own reason instead of automatically following the dictates of God or parents.

Similar strategies could be used to help teach children the basic principles of human communication and negotiation. For example, the teacher may devise a scenario for role playing, choosing a situation that will inevitably generate conflict and hence run the risk of making some children angry at the comments or behavior of others. At a certain point, Johnny becomes angry at Suzy, decides he doesn't want to play anymore, and starts to walk away. The teacher brings him back and encourages a discussion of Johnny's options. Johnny reveals that his parents always told him that if he ever felt angry at anyone he should walk away, thereby communicating to him that he should be afraid of his anger. In the following discussion Johnny learns about ways of expressing his angry feelings that enable him to continue to talk with the individual whose behavior has produced the feeling. Further discussions may lead Johnny to realize that he can keep the negotiation going until a satisfactory resolution of the conflict has been realized, with compromise on both sides.

This is, admittedly, a simplistic example. Moreover, programs of this sort could be mounted with properly trained teachers only if there was very close cooperation between the home and the school. Just as in the area of sex, parent education is as vital as the education of the child. If the father is a violent man who lashes out instinctively when angry or if Mother gives Father the silent treatment when she is angry at him, it would be difficult for the child to learn adaptive ways of handling anger. In other words, the parent would have to go back to school for the program to succeed with the child.

HUMANISM AND THE SOCIOPOLITICAL ARENA

Some humanists tend to comfort themselves with the myth that if we exercise enough patience, religion will eventually destroy itself. These inveterate optimists point to such things as the tension within the Roman Catholic Church on a wide variety of issues, or to the Jimmy Bakker scandal, as evidence that the institution called the Christian church will ultimately self-destruct. They fail to realize that shooting oneself in the foot is not the same thing as committing suicide. Such wishful thinking ignores the fact that the pope has many supporters within the Church. Even more important, if American Catholics were to break formally with Rome, as the English church did some 400 years ago, there is still nothing to suggest that this would prove damaging to the Body of Christ that is the Christian church. The church, in fact, could be said to have thrived on division and separations—from the great schisms of the eleventh century onward—in the manner of a giant pathogenic amoeba that multiples by cell division.

There is a good reason why humanists want to believe in the myth that a belief system as bizarre and anti-human as Christianity is bound to fall under the weight of time and human reason. Most of us have developed an antipathy toward institutions based largely on our experience with religious ones, and we do not eagerly take up the challenge of doing what we know we must. Until we realize that religion will not die a natural death and that we must develop into a political force to starve the dragon guarding the door of the future, there may be no future for our great-great grandchildren. In every community in the so-called Christian world, humanists must challenge religious influence in all areas of life. For every Christian pronouncement, from papal bulls downward, the humanist voice must be heard in response and refutation. Universities should set up programs in humanist studies in the same way that they have established women's studies. We need more humanist bookstores; newspapers must come to devote as much space to humanism as they do now to religion.

Above all, we need to establish more community humanist centers where people can be helped on the long, often painful, road from religious addiction to freethought. Many come only partway along the road, reluctant to take the final step into freedom. Others, who still call themselves Christian, admit, when pressed, to having given up the essential beliefs of Christianity even while clinging to a belief in "something out there." They continue to go to church, mouthing the prayers and singing the hymns that promote the very beliefs they claim to have rejected. To make matters worse, many of these people continue to subject their children to this kind of indoctrination on the mistaken assumption the child will learn morality from it all, without bothering to see how the experience is really affecting the child, or examining whether religion really does promote morality.

Rubbing shoulders with other people who are traveling the same road can be a useful experience; community humanist centers could, through lectures, readings, and group sessions, help people struggling in this way. Many "closet humanists" feel vaguely guilty about not going to church and have trouble relating to their church-going neighbors. They need some place they can call home, in which they can feel pride, not guilt, for throwing off the religious yoke, and where they can receive the support and encouragement to keep on the road toward humanism.

Christianity preaches that this world is a battleground in which holy men wage never-ending war against the forces of evil. We human beings are like a country in conflict, in which two rival powers are fighting for control. In order for this territory to be reclaimed by men and women, we must understand the rules of the game imposed on the human condition by the Christian religion. The views of philosopher Ludwig Feuerbach were discussed in chapter 2. According to Feuerbach, religious systems project the best human qualities onto the deity; these valued characteristics in human beings are then deemed to be mere reflections of the same qualities in the deity. Thus when an individual behaves immorally, it must never be related in any causal way to the Christian belief system, but must rather be an indication of a fall from grace. If a Christian behaves in a humane, moral manner, it must never be thought that this arises out of innate human decency, but is, rather, the result of Christian beliefs.

CONCLUSION

Religions—Christianity most of all—are the enemy of human morality. As we have seen throughout this book, many of Christianity's doctrinal beliefs work against the development of the full moral potential of human beings. It is ludicrous to believe that men and women can develop into moral beings by manipulating their guilt, treating them like small children, and urging them to be afraid of their natural impulses.

Those who set themselves up as the deity's interpreters form institutions that develop their own strategies, which are designed to expand and consolidate power over the believer. In the case of Christianity, these god-talking shepherds have been able to convince the sheep that they are innately evil and that "all good things come from God." The first step for the pilgrim on the road toward humanism is to understand this, "the great projection." The next step is to repudiate the destructive myth of innate evil.

"It is better to trust in the Lord than to put confidence in man" says psalm 108, verse 8. We have attempted to demonstrate that this belief, engrained as it is in the religious conciousness of Western society, has had a devastating impact on interpersonal relationships and human health. The medical profession, the pharmaceutical industry, and high-tech medicine are collectively blamed for the high costs of health care, some of which is well-deserved. However, no accusing fingers are ever pointed at the institution that promotes suffering as a valuable strategy, and whose doctrines have been shown to compromise human health in a variety of ways.

Can we ignore this fact much longer? There is no evidence that the modern versions of the Christian belief system, replete with "retrieval critique analysis," "embodiment theology," and other examples of "rectification," are any less destructive than the traditional one. The core doctrine remains the same.

Many humanists urge a less militant approach than is suggested here, arguing that people have as much right to follow their religious belief system as we humanists have to follow ours, and that they should not be criticized for it. Up to a point, this is a valid position, but one that warrants a closer look. If, as I have demonstrated in this book, Christian indoctrination is a form of mental and emotional abuse inflicted on innocent children, do we humanists have the moral right to remain silent about it? The state certainly plays an active role in preventing young people from becoming addicted to tobacco and alcohol (though not as successfully as many would like to see); does it not follow logically that the state might be expected to play a similar role in protecting young children from another form of toxic addiction?

There is an evolutionary process at work here. At one time, a "man's home was his castle," and the state had no right to intervene if a man chose to beat his children in obedience to the biblical injunction about sparing the rod and spoiling the child; or if he battered or raped his wife, since she was his property. Now the state takes a radically different view of all such forms of abuse, to the extent that health care professionals can be charged if they fail to report suspected instances of spouse or child abuse. Admittedly, in comparison with physical and sexual mistreatment, the matter of mental and emotional abuse is proving more difficult for the justice system to deal with; however, there are signs that these forms of maltreatment are gradually acquiring judicial legitimacy. Many humanists are in the forefront of the struggle to end physical and sexual molestation of children. How then can we remain sanguine about this other form of abuse?

Whatever we do, we must ensure that education, not legislation, is the strategy used to effect change. There must be no attempt to use the state to outlaw religion, even if Christianity has no compunction about using the state to extinguish other faith systems; however, we must be vigilant in order to prevent the state from using its power to suppress the humanist alternative. We believe that there can be no freedom *of* religion unless there is freedom *from* religion.

So long as Christian churches enjoy their tax-free status and other kinds of state support, Christian doctrine will continue to compromise our potential to work together to solve the problems threatening our global village. Only if Homo religiosus evolves into Homo sapiens can our species hope to survive. Surely it is time we, in the twentieth century, completed what others started at the time of the Renaissance.

NOTES

1. Bertrand Russell, *Why I Am Not a Christian* (London: Allen and Unwin, 1967), p. 42.

2. Paul Kurtz, *In Defense of Secular Humanism* (Buffalo, N.Y.: Prometheus Books, 1983), p. 23.

3. Stephen D. Mumford, *American Democracy and the Vatican: Population Growth and National Security* (Amherst, N.Y.: Humanist Press, 1984).

4. T. S. Eliot, "Four Quartets: East Coker," in *Selected Poems of T. S. Eliot* (London: Faber Paperbacks, 1963), p. 203.

5. Christopher Podmore, "Reflections on the Zundel and Keegstra Affairs," *Humanist in Canada* 18, no. 4 (Winter 1985/86): 75.

6. "Teacher Resigns Post amid Controversy," the (Hamilton, Ontario) *Spectator,* June 1, 1988, p. A5.

7. Stevi Jackson, *Childhood and Sexuality* (Oxford: Basil Blackwell, 1982), p. 152.

Bibliography

Allegro, John M. *The Dead Sea Scrolls and the Christian Myth*. Buffalo, N.Y.: Prometheus Books, 1984.

Alvarez, A. *The Savage God: A Study in Suicide*. New York: Random House, 1972.

Armstrong, Karen. *The Gospel according to Woman*. London: Elm Tree Books, 1986.

Batson, C. Daniel, and W. Larry Ventis. *The Religious Experience*. New York: Oxford University Press, Inc., 1982.

Bibby, Reginald. *Fragmented Gods: The Poverty and Potential of Religion in Canada*. Toronto: Irwin Publishing, 1987.

Bullough, Vern L. *Sexual Variance in Society and History*. Chicago: The University of Chicago Press, 1976.

Bullough, Vern L., and James Brundage. *Sexual Practices and the Medieval Church*. Buffalo, N.Y.: Prometheus Books, 1982.

Butler, Sandra. *Conspiracy of Silence: The Trauma of Incest*. San Francisco: New Glide Publications, 1978.

Cohen, Edmund D. *The Mind of the Bible-Believer*. Buffalo, N.Y.: Prometheus Books, 1986.

Daly, Mary. *The Church and the Second Sex*. Boston: Beacon Press, 1985.

Ellis, Albert. *The Case against Religion: A Psychotherapist's View,* and *The Case Against Religiosity*. Austin, Tex.: American Atheist Press, n.d.

Feinberg, Abraham. *Sex and the Pulpit*. Toronto: Methuen Publications, 1981.

Feuerbach, Ludwig. *The Essence of Christianity*. Trans. George Eliot. Buffalo, N.Y.: Prometheus Books, 1989.

Gascoigne, Bamber. *The Christians*. London: Granada Publishing, 1978.

Greeley, Roger, ed. *The Best of Robert Ingersoll.* Buffalo, N.Y.: Prometheus Books, 1983.

Jackson, Stevi. *Childhood and Sexuality.* Oxford: Basil Blackwell, 1982.

Hoffmann, R. Joseph, and Gerald A. Larue, eds. *Jesus in History and Myth.* Buffalo, N.Y.: Prometheus Books, 1986.

Kramer, Heinrich, and James Sprenger. *The Malleus Maleficarum.* New York: Dover Publications, 1971.

Kurtz, Paul. *In Defense of Secular Humanism.* Buffalo, N.Y.: Prometheus Books, 1983.

———, ed. *Building a World Community: Humanism in the 21st Century.* Buffalo, N.Y.: Prometheus Books, 1989.

Lader, Lawrence. *Politics, Power and the Church.* New York: Macmillan Publishing Company, 1987.

Masson, Jeffrey Moussaieff. *The Assault on Truth: Freud's Suppression of the Seduction Theory.* New York: Farrar, Straus and Giroux, 1984.

Miller, Alice. *For Your Own Good.* New York: Farrar, Straus and Giroux, 1990.

Miller, William A. *Why Do Christians Break Down.* Minneapolis, Minn.: Augsburg Publishing House, 1973.

Mumford, Stephen D. *American Democracy and the Vatican: Population Growth and National Security.* Amherst, N.Y.: Humanist Press, 1984.

Peck, M. Scott. *The Road Less Travelled.* New York: Simon and Schuster, 1978.

Richardson, Alan. *Creeds in the Making.* Philadelphia: Fortress Press, 1981.

Rosenberg, Stuart E. *The Christian Problem: A Jewish View.* Toronto: Deneau Publishers, 1986.

Russell, Bertrand. *Why I Am Not a Christian.* London: Unwin Paperbacks, 1967.

Smith, George H. *Atheism: The Case against God.* Buffalo, N.Y.: Prometheus Books, 1979.

Stein, Gordon, ed. *An Anthology of Atheism and Rationalism.* Buffalo, N.Y.: Prometheus Books, 1980.

Stern, E. Mark, ed. *Psychotherapy and the Religiously Committed Patient.* New York: Haworth Press, Inc., 1985.

Sutherland, Charles. *Disciples of Destruction: The Religious Origins of War and Terrorism.* Buffalo, N.Y.: Prometheus Books, 1987.

Seligman, Martin E. P. *Helplessness: On Depression, Development and Death.* San Francisco: W. H. Freeman and Company, 1975.

Tannahill, Reay. *Sex in History.* New York: Stein and Day, 1980.

Thomas à Kempis. *The Imitation of Christ.* Chicago: Moody Press, 1980.

Watters, Wendell W. *Compulsory Parenthood: The Truth about Abortion.* Toronto: McClelland and Stewart, 1976.

Index